The International Library of Psychology

PERSONALITY AND THE
FRONTAL LOBES

Founded by C. K. Ogden

The International Library of Psychology

ABNORMAL AND CLINICAL PSYCHOLOGY
In 19 Volumes

PERSONALITY AND THE FRONTAL LOBES

An Investigation of the Psychological Effects of Different Types of Leucotomy

ASENATH PETRIE

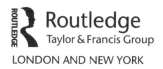

Routledge
Taylor & Francis Group

LONDON AND NEW YORK

First published in 1952 by
Routledge and Kegan Paul Ltd
2 Park Square, Milton Park, Abingdon, Oxfordshire OX14 4RN
711 Third Avenue, New York, NY 10017

First issued in paperback 2014

Routledge is an imprint of the Taylor and Francis Group, an informa business

British Library Cataloguing in Publication Data
A CIP catalogue record for this book
is available from the British Library

Personality and the Frontal Lobes
ISBN 978-0415-20932-8
Abnormal and Clinical Psychology: 19 Volumes
ISBN 0415-21123-9
The International Library of Psychology: 204 Volumes
ISBN 0415-19132-7
Printed and bound by CPI Antony Rowe, Eastbourne

ISBN 13: 978-1-138-88239-3 (pbk)
ISBN 13: 978-0-415-20932-8 (hbk)

' I cou'd be mighty foolish, and fancy
myself mighty witty; reason still keeps
its Throne— but it nods a little, that's all.'

FARQUHAR, GEORGE (1678–1707)

CONTENTS

CONTENTS

INTRODUCTION

IT is recognised that the brain is the physical background of intellect. That an alteration to an individual's brain will alter both temperament and character is less well assured. Yet when the neural connections in the front of the brain, that is, in the frontal lobes, are severed that is what in fact happens. The individual shows a dramatic change in personality, in temperament, character and ability.

Because such alterations in personality can be induced, a surgical operation on the frontal lobes is carried out in an attempt to alleviate the condition of individuals affected with certain mental illnesses; and recently to relieve intractable pain which proves incapable of relief by other methods of treatment. In this operation, called prefrontal leucotomy, the main connections between the frontal lobes and the thalamus are severed.

This book sets out to present the results of an investigation into the effect on character, temperament and intellectual aspects of personality induced respectively by four different types of leucotomy. These various approaches were tried with the aim, expressed by Professor Adrian in 1948, of arriving at a procedure which caused the maximum reduction in anxiety but the minimum of irresponsibility in the patient. In addition to this clinical application, it is hoped that the results may be of assistance in the diagnosis of injury to the frontal lobes in war casualties and peacetime accidents. Knowledge of the nature of the deficit caused by this operation also indicates which aspects of personality should be stressed in a rehabilitation programme prepared both for patients so injured and those who have undergone the operation of leucotomy.

The study of the effect of lesions in this area of the brain may indeed have wider socio-biological interest, because even if there is not universal agreement with Penfield's (1950) statement that the frontal lobes are 'the only part of the (human) brain that distinguishes it from a chimpanzee', it is agreed that they do constitute one of the major differences between the two.

Prefrontal leucotomy has been used since 1935, but the early patients selected for operation were so ill mentally that it was difficult to ascertain what exactly was happening to the personality as a result of the operation. More recently some of the patients operated on have been severe neurotics who in comparison with the patients in mental hospitals were so nearly normal that they presented a unique opportunity to try to ascertain by objective tests, with which considerable advances have been made in the last few years, what did actually happen to the individual's personality when incisions were made in the frontal lobes of his brain.

The material collected in this study has been subjected to statistical analysis by independent computors who were unaware of the relevance of the various scores to this investigation and are not open to the suspicion of any *a priori* views. I am greatly indebted to the Scientific Computing Service and especially to Dr. Gillis who carried out this work.

The text has been kept as free as possible of statistical details so that those uninterested in this aspect of the subject should have no difficulty in understanding the main trends of the deductions. Chapter V, however, may cause a little difficulty to those unfamiliar with statistics. The figures in this chapter can, if need be, be neglected without much detriment to the main argument.

It is hoped that the investigations here detailed illustrate the serious repercussions of leucotomy and may thus encourage the continued exercise of the utmost caution in its use.

ACKNOWLEDGMENTS

THIS work could not have been completed without the help and co-operation of very many people. It is lack of space, not of gratitude, which prevents my mentioning all individually.

It was Dr. Desmond Curran, Head of the Department of Psychiatry, St. George's Hospital, London, who, in 1946, suggested to me the desirability of an investigation into the effects of leucotomy. I am not only indebted to him for the facilities with which I was subsequently provided, but his support and guidance during the five years I spent on this work have been of the greatest assistance. I am grateful also to Mr. Wylie McKissock whose skill enabled me to compare the effect of different types of operation.

It gives me much pleasure to express my indebtedness to Professor Aubrey Lewis whose help and encouragement have been a continuous inspiration; to Professor Alfred Meyer for invaluable assistance on anatomical aspects which he alone was in a position to provide; and to his associates, Mrs. Beck and Dr. Turner McLardy, more especially for the diagrams in Chapter I.

I have to thank Sir Paul Mallinson, Dr. Louis Minski, Dr. D. N. Parfit, Dr. Maurice Partridge and Dr. Thomas Tennent for permitting me to examine their cases; Dr. Fleminger, Dr. Ford and Dr. Liddell whose case notes have been of great assistance to me; and particularly Dr. Humphry Osmond who was responsible for the organisation of the clinical assessments and who has helped with other aspects of the work. I am indebted to Sisters Cooper and Rae of the Psychiatric Wards who have assisted me in many ways.

I also had the great advantage of the help of Dr. Douglas Robson who, in his dual capacity as psychiatrist and psychologist, has read through the whole of this manuscript as well as giving generously of his leisure to assist with many different aspects of the investigation.

ACKNOWLEDGMENTS

My indebtedness to my colleague, Dr. H. J. Eysenck, Reader in Psychology at the Institute of Psychiatry, London University, for his guidance and help in all stages of the work is very great. Among other psychologists whose help I would like gratefully to record are Dr. H. T. Himmelweit of the London School of Economics, Dr. Johanna Krout of Chicago, U.S.A., and Dr. S. Crown, of the Maudsley Hospital, who read the proofs.

The Board of Governors of St. George's Hospital have kindly voted a grant towards the cost of the statistical analysis; Mr. T. H. Constable, the House Governor, has smoothed out difficulties in whatever ways lay open to him.

It is difficult for me adequately to thank Dr. R. N. Salaman, F.R.S., who read through the whole of the manuscript and made invaluable suggestions regarding the presentation of material. From him I have learned how much the discipline of one science may be enriched by contact with another. Not less am I indebted to Mr. and Mrs. A. Shonfield for their criticisms and suggestions.

Finally I wish to express my gratitude to the most long-suffering and patient of all, Mrs. Winifred Hunt, who has given me irreplaceable secretarial help and has typed this manuscript in her well-earned leisure. It is due to her ability that the final passage of this book to the press has been attained.

ASENATH PETRIE

Department of Psychology,
  University of Pennsylvania,
    Philadelphia, U.S.A.
October, 1951.

CHAPTER ONE

HISTORY OF THE OPERATION OF LEUCOTOMY
AND OUTLINE OF INVESTIGATIONS
TO BE REPORTED IN THIS BOOK

ONE of the first cases in which a personality change was observed to follow on an injury to the brain was reported in 1835. Nobele, in a Belgian medical journal, described a psychotic patient who attempted suicide by shooting himself through the head. He nearly succeeded; the bullet did penetrate his skull though it failed to kill him, but afterwards his mental illness had disappeared. During the next hundred years much physiological work on the cerebral cortex was done, but it was not until the thirties of this century that Moniz of Lisbon carried out the first operation on the frontal lobes in an attempt to alleviate mental illness. He published his results in 1936.

The most anterior portion of the frontal lobes, the prefrontal cortex, is scarcely represented at all in lower mammals and, where present, never approaches in development that of the human brain. It was usually thought that this must be concerned with man's 'higher thoughts', and various suggestions were made as to the changes which group themselves under this heading.

Its presence in apes made certain experiments possible; indeed, the report of one piece of research carried out by Jacobsen with chimpanzees in 1936 is believed to have stimulated Moniz to develop his ideas with regard to the use of the operation in human beings. One of the chimpanzees had previously been extraordinarily disturbed when she made a mistake in the course of an attempt to open puzzle boxes that contained food. After the operation she was making more mistakes but displaying great calm.

P.F.L.—I   I

Our knowledge of the effect of interference with the frontal lobes in man until then was based on observations of the effect of accidents involving these areas, or of changes following the removal of tumours. It was noted, for example, that when a perfectly normal man, Phineas Gage, had his frontal lobes damaged through an accident with a crowbar, he had changed to such an extent that 'he was no longer Gage'. It was not just that he had a scar or was not so clever at solving a problem, but the 'aroma' of his personality was different (Harlow, 1848). Other cases were subsequently described of frontal lesions leading to alterations of character and moral behaviour (Welt, 1888; Bruns, 1897).

The innovation of Moniz—a brain operation to relieve mental illness and causing a dramatic change in personality— did not go uncriticised. But Moniz continued to use and develop his frontal lobe operation, and it was pursued by Drs. Freeman and Watts in the United States of America. The results of the work improved as more satisfactory methods of operating were developed. After the publication of the first book on the effects of this operation (Freeman and Watts, 1942), it was increasingly widely used, both in the States and in Europe, on psychotics, neurotics and finally for the relief of intractable pain.

What is the Effect of Leucotomy?

Leucotomy, as the operation is called in Europe, is the most drastic physical treatment carried out in psychiatry, so that the importance of an accurate assessment of its results can scarcely be overstressed. Until recently such assessments as have been made were chiefly in the form of clinical descriptions. Thus there are reports of greater complacency, tactlessness, self-will, less self-criticism, reserve and shyness, lessening of self-consciousness, of awareness of feelings of others and reliability, increased shallowness, less emotional sensitivity and a loss in subtlety and insight into subjects' own mental mechanism.[1]

---

[1] There are numerous contributions and reviews of the clinical aspects of leucotomy. It is impossible to refer to all of these, but among the many which contributed to the planning of this investigation in 1947 were those of Brickner (1936), Rylander (1939), Dax and Radley Smith (1943), Freeman and Watts (1944) and Berliner et al. (1945). Some other references are presented in Appendix E.

Many of these clinical descriptions are of inestimable value and many of them include, in addition to the impressions of the doctor, those of the family and associates of the patient. But it is inherent in such impressions that they vary with the observer; it was therefore important to add to these clinical impressions the check of scientific measurements carried out under conditions which can be repeated in an identical form by other investigators and which do not depend upon the subjective estimate of the observer. This is what has been attempted.

We were primarily interested in obtaining information from objective tests as to the nature of the changes following on this operation. In addition, we were interested in whether, by means of such objective tests, it could be demonstrated that a less severe or different type of operation to that commonly used would produce different results. It was hoped, moreover, that we might be able to throw some light on the phenomena associated with improvement after the operation. Present also was the wish, rather than the hope, that such investigations might make some small contribution towards the understanding of the function of the intact frontal lobes in man.

Some thousands of patients have undergone prefrontal leucotomy in this country between 1940 and 1950, but most of these people were so severely ill mentally that no adequate measurement of personality could have been carried out, and therefore no reliable estimate could have been made as to the effect of the operation. Investigators in the past who have worked with psychotics undergoing leucotomy have been confronted with the difficulties arising from having too many unknown variables. The patients used for the investigations to be reported in this book were probably as near the normal as any likely to be operated upon. They were in the main neurotics, and the operation was carried out to relieve them of their neurosis. Their personalities were so well preserved that they could co-operate through the many hours of testing necessitated by this investigation. In comparison with psychotics who are usually subjected to this treatment it seemed probable that these patients would provide us with much more reliable information as to its effect.

Such objective investigations as had been carried out previously appear to have certain serious limitations in addition to

3

the severity of the mental illness of the patients examined.[1] One of these was the almost complete preoccupation until fairly recent times with the attempt to show changes on intelligence tests. This practice is related to the history of the development of methods of mental measurements, in which it appeared to be of more immediate practical importance to measure the intellectual ability of an individual than his character and temperament. This was partly due to the pressing problems of separating those of low-grade intelligence who could not profit from teaching designed for the more intelligent and who acted as a brake on the speed at which the latter were allowed to learn. Thus methods of measuring intelligence were developed before those measuring temperament and character, and it was natural that the effect of an injury on the frontal lobes, said to be concerned with the higher functions of men, should be measured by these tests of intelligence. The absence of marked effects on mental ability, as measured by these intelligence tests, was, not surprisingly, felt to be puzzling. The patients were manifestly different as a result of leucotomy. This was the opinion of the doctors, the nurses, the family and friends of the patient. Yet intellectually they were relatively the same. What was this change? Was it an illusion? Or were the measurements perhaps inadequate? As one writer on frontal lobe operations has said, 'one common criticism of scientific methods as applied to the present sphere is that it has not yielded quantitative support of phenomena which anyone, using merely observation, can easily perceive. Since scientific tests answer only the questions they have been designed to ask it is, of course, possible that the proper tests have not been devised' (Mettler, 1949).

The development of objective methods of personality measurements

In recent years a considerable amount of intensive work has been carried out on the measurement of those aspects of personality which are in the sphere of temperament or character rather than of intelligence. Such work has been stimulated by the experiences of the Services during the war. It was apparent that a high intelligence level was not sufficient by itself to deter-

[1] In view of the number of psychological investigations on leucotomy patients that have been reported and the diversity of approaches to the problem, a brief survey of such work is presented separately in Appendix E.

mine the suitability or otherwise of a man in a key position; that orectic aspects of personality needed to be taken into account. and that from the practical viewpoint it was important, if at all possible, to weed out the potential breakdowns before they occurred. In order to do this, adequate methods of measuring personality had to be found.

The intensive development of objective methods of personality measurements in England since 1940 has taken place under the leadership of Dr. Eysenck and his associates, first at Mill Hill Emergency Hospital and after the war at the Maudsley Hospital (Eysenck, 1947). Eysenck argued that measurement in the field of personality is impossible until the dimensions along which such measurements can be made are known. To arrive at such dimensions he first of all utilised the ratings by psychiatrists of the history, symptoms, diagnoses, treatment and disposal of 700 neurotic soldiers (Eysenck, 1944A). These items were subjected to the mathematical process known as factorial analysis. The aim of factorial analysis is to discover the smallest number of independent variables which will adequately describe and classify personality traits. It is not proposed to enter into details of the technicalities of this method, nor its rationale. It will suffice for purposes of this exposition to state that factorial analysis enables one to recognise those ratings (or tests) which tend to cohere together and define a dimension of personality.

Eysenck's study resulted in the identification of two personality factors. Subject to various reservations, these factors were labelled 'neuroticism' and 'extraversion-introversion'. Both of these dimensions were closely related to similar factors previously described in normal and neurotic subjects by many workers. For example, Cattell (1946A, 1950), working with objective tests and ratings in the States, had arrived at factors he has called 'C' and 'F' respectively. These are for our purpose identical with what Eysenck calls 'neuroticism' and 'introversion'; throughout this book we will be using Eysenck's terminology. In addition to the two main dimensions being corroborated by other contemporary psychologists, the evidence pointed to their being identical with the theoretical concepts of Janet (1903), Jung (1923), McDougall (1926), Luria (1932) and Pavlov (1941).

The isolation of these factors appeared to suggest two dimensions of personality along which measurement might usefully be undertaken. An effort was therefore made to discover those objective tests which would make measurement of these dimensions possible. A group of such objective personality tests was found to be related to the dimension of 'neuroticism'; a further group of tests was found to be related to the dimension 'extraversion-introversion'. Thus greater ideomotor suggestibility, poorer manual dexterity, slower speed of writing and so on were found to be related to 'neuroticism'; and greater accuracy and slower speed, preoccupation with the past rather than the present and the future, low rating of sex humour were found to be related to 'introversion' as opposed to 'extraversion'.

Considerable experimental work has been carried out using these objective tests on a variety of subjects (Eysenck, 1947; Pichot, 1949); including, for example, former prisoners-of-war (Himmelweit *et al.*, 1946), patients in a wartime neurosis centre (Petrie, 1948A), mental defectives (Brady, 1948), medical students (Petrie, 1948B), epileptics (M. D. Eysenck, 1950), student nurses (Petrie and Powell, 1950 and 1951) and normal and neurotic children (Himmelweit and Petrie, 1951). All these studies have supplied further evidence regarding these two dimensions and the associated objective measurements.

FRONTAL LOBE OPERATIONS AND OBJECTIVE PERSONALITY MEASUREMENTS

Such objective investigations of personality changes after leucotomy as have been carried out in the past seem to have been largely empirical. A fair proportion of the tests used were selected more or less at random and without any hypothesis as to their relevance to the problem. There are, however, practical advantages in first trying to enunciate a clear-cut hypothesis as to the changes likely to be caused by the operation and select the tests so as to verify or disprove it. The investigations to be reported in this book are an attempt to do this.

A study of the literature of the 'new' personality resulting from the Standard posterior operation, the most usual form of leucotomy in this country, led to the formulation of the following hypotheses:

6

that alterations would occur in three main dimensions of personality—degree of neuroticism, degree of introversion and degree of intelligence;

that the direction of the change would be a decrease in neuroticism, a movement away from the introverted end of the scale towards the extraverted end and a decrease in certain aspects of intelligence;

that after a more anterior operation the extent of these changes would be less, whilst the pattern remained the same.

Investigations to be described in this book were designed to test these hypotheses; tests were therefore used which have been shown to be related to the dimensions. In addition to tests related to neuroticism and to extraversion, a number of different types of intelligence tests were used in order to ascertain whether any special aspects of intelligence were affected by the operation.

Although the investigation was designed to test these hypotheses, it was realised that incidental information collected might prove of value; and an attempt was made to design some further tests that would measure changes that had been described in the literature.

Patients undergoing four different types of operation were examined, before and after the operation; viz. a group of patients who were undergoing the Standard type of operation; another group who were undergoing a more anterior operation than that commonly practised; and two further groups who were operated on one side only—a unilateral anterior operation on either the left or right frontal lobe. It was hoped that as four different types of operation were being compared, the changes found on objective tests might indicate by which method some of the undesired and undesirable effects of the operation could be avoided. Moreover, if one could predict the probability of the nature and extent of the changes in personality following on each one, it might bring us nearer to the goal of fitting the operation to the individual personality.

Patients

The patients on whom we are reporting were, with but a few exceptions, seen at St. George's Hospital, London, a general teaching hospital, and were operated on at its Psychiatric Unit at the Atkinson Morley Hospital. None of these patients were certifiable, the vast majority of them being severe neurotics.[1] They were primarily obsessional, anxiety or depressed patients and some had hysterical symptoms. The percentage in the diagnostic groups is given in detail when presenting the results of each investigation, but it can be stated here that there was no significant difference in the distribution of the diagnostic categories in the main groups we have studied.

There was no selection of the patients subjected to each of the various types of operation. In every case a conference took place after the patient had been an in-patient in hospital for a period sufficiently long to assess the prognosis without leucotomy. At this conference with their chief assistants, registrars and nursing sisters, the physicians decided whether or not to recommend the operation. This decision was nearly always based on there being no reasonable alternative treatment which would meet the urgent social needs of the patient. Four of the patients came from Belmont Hospital, where a comparable form of selection took place under the supervision of Dr. Louis Minski.

Within a certain period all patients recommended for leucotomy were subjected to the Standard type of operation. During a further period all patients were subjected to the Rostral operation. Some patients were given a unilateral operation only, and an attempt was made to alternate the left and right sides.

With regard to one aspect, both Crown (1951), using psychotic patients, and myself, using neurotic patients, had similar difficulties. This was the impossibility of matching our operated group with a control group which was comparable in the relevant variables. We started by testing individuals who were thought to be adequate controls. One of two developments took place in each case: either it was decided that they were to be leucotomised and thus became part of our experimental population or, after further investigation, it was found that they were quite unsuitable for leucotomy and quite unlike the patient who was, and thus they became unsuitable as a matched control.

It is worth mentioning that the one significant difference

[1] The records of patients who, on reassessment after the operation, were diagnosed as psychotics or who needed mental care have been excluded from this analysis.

8

found in a group of patients undergoing operations in the Columbia-Greystone Project (Garrison, 1949) could not be evaluated against an attempted control group; that is, they found that the operated population differed to such an extent initially from the control population with regard to anxieties and complaints that any arguments of a change due to the operation needed to be based on the scores of the operated group alone.

In the investigation reported in this book the results after the Standard operation have been chosen as a base line in comparing the three other types of operation with one another. The justification for this lies in the clear-cut agreement between the pattern of changes at the early and later investigation of the Standard, and the manner in which the remaining data bear out these findings.

The Operations

All patients were operated on by the same neurosurgeon, Mr. Wylie McKissock.

Changes in patients who have undergone four main types of operation will be reported. Firstly the results of the Standard operation, the one which is most frequently used, will be dealt with. This is a closed bilateral operation and is the most posterior of those described. This operation is performed through a trephine hole in the skull on each side.

Mr. McKissock describes the Standard operation as follows:

'I have in general taken a point 3 cm. behind the lateral margin of the orbit and 5–6 cm. above the zygoma as the centre of my 2–3 cm. skin incision. The incision is made down to the bone, and a self-retaining retractor inserted firmly to give a wide exposure and a bloodless field. A 1 cm. burr-hole is then cut in the line of the coronal suture and a cruciform incision made in the dura.

'The instrument used for the section of the white matter is the least damaging of all—an ordinary brain needle, with a side eyelet just short of the blunt point, and a close-fitting stylet. This is introduced in such a direction as to pass close in front of the anterior horn of the ventricle to a depth sufficient to be just clear of the grey matter of the inner aspect of the frontal lobe.

The stylet is withdrawn and the needle made to pivot about the point of entrance through the dura so that the blunt inner extremity travels upwards towards the superior surface of the frontal lobe. As the point is made to travel upwards the needle is pushed more deeply into the brain so that the line of the section runs parallel with the falx and does not, as it otherwise would, become steadily more distant from it. When the needle has reached sufficiently close to the upper surface of the hemisphere it is withdrawn and reintroduced along the original line in order to deal with those fibres running from the lower part of the frontal pole; on this occasion the point of the needle is made to travel downwards, again parallel with the falx, and is then brought laterally across the anterior fossa roughly in the same vertical plane as the lesser wing of the sphenoid, until it reaches a point just short of the lateral aspect of the skull. During this part of the section the needle is progressively withdrawn for fear of damaging the grey matter of the orbital surface of the frontal pole.

'A wet patty is then left in the opening in the bone whilst the performance is repeated on the opposite frontal lobe.' (McKissock, 1943.)

The second type of operation, the Rostral, is more anterior than the Standard and is an open bilateral operation. The Rostral operation is carried out through a pair of burr-holes under direct vision. It cuts most of the convexity fibres and leaves the orbital aspect relatively free, areas 9 and 10 being primarily involved.

'Through a pair of burr-holes on either side of the midline just in front of the coronal suture he incised the superior frontal convolution transversely and then sucked out a thin layer of the white matter down to the orbital plane. He made it 2–2·25 cm. wide and 6–8 cm. deep so that it was an extremely limited type of section. As it was done under direct vision, any interference with the function of the brain on either side was prevented.' (McKissock, 1949.)

The two remaining types of operation were carried out on one side only. These were unilateral Rostral operations on the left and right side respectively. Each of these is an open operation carried out through a burr-hole under direct vision.

OUTLINE OF INVESTIGATION

We propose to refer in this text to the Standard as the posterior operation, the Rostral as the anterior operation and the unilateral as left and right anterior operations respectively. The plane of each operation has been indicated in *Diagrams I, II* and *III*. It will be noted that the difference between the plane of the two types of operation is substantial and may reach approximately 50% of the prefrontal region.

OUTLINE OF INVESTIGATION

All patients were examined before and after the operation. In the case of the posterior Standard operation we saw each patient approximately two weeks before the operation, three months after the operation and again nine months after the operation. We hoped thus to obtain an indication of the reliability of the first changes noted and some evidence as to whether alterations in behaviour took place over the longer period.

The anterior open operation, the Rostral, was followed up at an interval of approximately six months, so that each patient was seen approximately two weeks before the operation and six months afterwards.

Various considerations determined the choice of these intervals. We were anxious to wait a sufficient time after the operation for the results to be reasonably representative of the stable condition of the post-leucotomy patient. It was realised that if the testing was carried out very soon after the operation, although it might present us with very interesting data regarding the traumatic effect of the incision, it would not give us a picture of the post-leucotomy patient.

We were guided in the choice of the interval before retesting in the first place by psychiatric opinion and the findings from electroencephalographic studies. Curran's and Guttman's (1943) advice regarding the disturbances of personality after cerebral injury and the time that should elapse before a prognosis can be reliably made is 'no opinion as to the final outcome should be expressed before two or three months after the injury have elapsed.' It has, moreover, been shown that the abnormal electroencephalographic waves after prefrontal leucotomy return to a normal pattern after one to three months (Cohn, 1945). Our first investigation after the operation was,

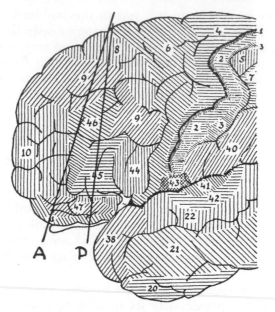

Diagram I.—LATERAL VIEW OF THE FRONTAL LOBE

A is the plane of the anterior Rostral incision.
P is the plane of the posterior Standard incision.
Superimposed on Brodman's cytoarchitectonic map.

therefore, carried out at an interval of approximately three months. When the results showed that some changes became more accentuated after a longer period, we increased the interval before the first retest to approximately six months.

The identical tests were given before and after the operation. Every attempt was made to ensure that the conditions were the same in each of the investigations. Each patient was given a wide and varied group of personality and intelligence tests; the personality tests included those which had been shown to be related to neuroticism, those which had been shown to be related to extraversion and introversion, and some of general interest whose relationship to these two dimensions has not, as yet, been clarified.

The results on each test are reported separately, but they are grouped in accordance with the main dimensions to which they are related. A comparison was made between scores before and

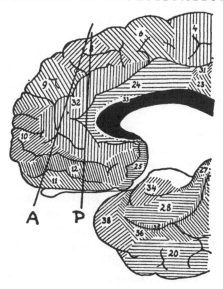

Diagram II.—MEDIAN VIEW OF THE FRONTAL LOBE

A is the plane of the anterior Rostral incision.
P is the plane of the posterior Standard incision.
Superimposed on Brodman's cytoarchitectonic map.

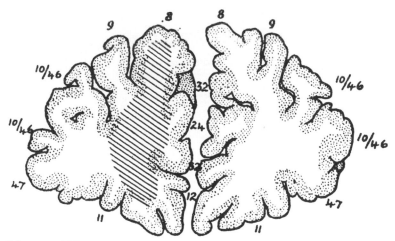

Diagram III.—CORONAL SECTION THROUGH THE FRONTAL
POLES AT THE LEVEL INDICATED AS A IN DIAGRAMS I AND II

The area involved in the unilateral Rostral operation is shaded.

13

after the operation. Such differences as were found between these two scores were subjected to statistical tests of significance. With certain exceptions, which will be indicated, only those changes will be reported where the probability is 19 to 1 against their having arisen by chance; that is, where, according to Fisher's 't' test,[1] the probability of such an event happening is less than 0·05.

The effect of the posterior Standard operation on personality will be reported in Chapters II and III. For the sake of convenience we are reporting orectic—those appertaining to temperament and character—and intellectual aspects separately. The effect of the anterior Rostral operation and the unilateral operations is described in Chapter IV. In Chapter V we will compare the effects of the various operations and consider the personality scores as related to clinical improvement. An attempt to synthesise these findings is made in Chapter VI. Details of tests, statistics, examples of patients' productions and case histories are to be found in the Appendices.

[1] Fisher's 't' test is a test of significance suitable for smaller numbers of subjects and is essentially equivalent to the critical ratio.

CHAPTER TWO

THE EFFECT OF POSTERIOR STANDARD LEUCOTOMY ON TEMPERAMENT AND CHARACTER

THIS chapter is mainly concerned with a description of the changes in temperament and character found after the blind Standard posterior operation.[1] The effects of this operation on intelligence and intellectual functioning will be dealt with in Chapter III. These two aspects of personality are of course separated in this way merely for the sake of convenience; they are continually interacting and are almost inextricably interwoven.

The patients were seen on three occasions—before the operation and twice after the operation. The first investigation took place approximately two weeks before the operation. The average interval between the operation and the second investigation was three months and that between the operation and the third investigation was nine months.[2]

The Patients

The data are based on changes in twenty-seven patients subjected to the Standard operation. Initially the pre-operative performance of twenty patients was compared with their performance three months after leucotomy. Later on four of these original twenty patients were not available. But as the investigations had been continued on incoming patients, the scores of

[1] The operation itself was described in Chapter I.

[2] Owing to administrative difficulties it was not possible to see all the patients after the operation at an interval of exactly three months. The range of this interval, however, was between two months and five months for the second investigation and between eight months and twelve months for the third investigation. The differences found can only have been attenuated as a result of this variation in time.

four 'new' patients were available for inclusion in the nine months' analysis, which was thus again a comparison of the pre-operative and post-operative performance of twenty patients. All of the patients in this second analysis, therefore, were tested on three separate occasions—before, and three months and nine months after the operation. The scores of patients who were included in both the three months' and nine months' analysis have been used to estimate the effects of the passage of time after the operation on personality. Three patients on whom data are incomplete have supplied examples of intellectual changes quoted in Chapter III and the Appendices.

In the whole group there were twenty-one women and six men. In both the retests, at three months and at nine months, which have been analysed for twenty patients, there are five men and fifteen women. Seventeen of the patients were married; the remaining ten were unmarried.

The patients had been given the usual forms of treatment— that is, psychotherapy and some types of physical treatment electric shock, narco-analysis and in some cases modified insulin, prior to the operation. The decision to operate was made by the physicians in charge after considering the prognosis without such treatment and the probability of the personality of the patient being such as to respond to leucotomy. The same criteria for the selection of patients has been used with regard to all groups studied.

The diagnostic grouping of the patients was as follows:

Of those included in the three months' analysis five (25%) were obsessionals, five (25%) were cases of depression, three (15%) were anxiety cases, one (5%) was hysterical and six (30%) were of mixed diagnosis, including one alcohol addict and one case of depersonalisation.

Of those included in the nine months' analysis seven (35%) were obsessionals, four (20%) were cases of depression, two (10%) were anxiety cases, two (10%) were hysterical and five (25%) were of mixed diagnosis.

In each group four of the five male patients were obsessionals and one was of mixed diagnosis.

Most of the patients had been in hospital for only a few weeks before the operation was carried out. A few had been in hospital before and had returned after an interval, but there had not been a long period of hospitalisation before the operation as is nearly always the case in groups of psychotics undergoing leucotomy. After the operation all patients remained in hospital for a minimum of four weeks; some with unfortunate home circumstances remained longer. In addition, a period of convalescence of four to six weeks was usually arranged before returning home or resuming work. The patients, moreover, had the benefit of the psychiatric social workers' untiring efforts on their behalf.

The average age of patients in the first investigation was 41·5 years (range 23 to 67); in the second 40·5 years (range 23 to 67). The average intelligence is represented by Wechsler I.Q. 105·9 (range 75 to 133) for patients in the first investigation and I.Q. 109·3 (range 75 to 133) for patients in the second investigation.

Three of the patients were university graduates. Eight had attended secondary school and three of these in addition had technical training. Five had technical training after an elementary education. The remaining ten had attended elementary school only.

The patients included one man who after the operation had gone back to work as a minister of religion, and others as a teacher in a secondary school, a bank cashier, an assistant nurse, a manager of an insurance company, an optician, a radio engineer and a bookseller. There were also two shorthand-typists and several housewives who resumed their duties at home. Some of the latter had previously been clerical workers, shopkeepers, telephonists and domestic workers. Only one of the twenty-seven patients was considered to be worse after the operation.[1]

Statistical Analysis of Scores

The standard of significance adopted throughout this work is that a finding would have occurred less than once in twenty times by chance (probability 0·05 using Fisher's 't' test). However, changes which do not reach this level have occasionally been reported, particularly when they are corroborated by the general trend or throw light on clinical descriptions in the

[1] See Chapter V.

literature; but these 'suggestive' changes have always been mentioned as such.

Tables and statistical details (mean difference, standard deviation of difference, critical ratio and probability) will be found in Appendix B at the end of the book.

Personality Tests Chosen

In the previous chapter were described the two dimensions of personality that have been identified and referred to by Eysenck (1947) as 'neuroticism' and 'extraversion-introversion'. It was also stated that a number of objective tests were found to be related to these dimensions, so that, for example, in the case of the factor 'neuroticism', individuals at the neurotic end of the scale were differentiated from those at the non-neurotic end by scores on a group of objective tests.

The hypothesis that was formulated regarding the personality changes following on leucotomy involved these two dimensions —it was suggested that there was a decrease in neuroticism and a decrease in introversion—as well as in certain aspects of intelligence. To investigate this hypothesis a number of tests related to each of these dimensions have been used.

In addition to the measurements chosen to test this hypothesis I have designed and used certain additional tests in order to tap other areas of personality in which changes are suggested in the literature.

THE DIMENSION OF NEUROTICISM: ASSOCIATED MEASUREMENTS

The following traits have been shown to be related to the dimension of neuroticism:

1. *Suggestibility*—the neurotic is more suggestible (Eysenck, 1944B; Petrie, 1948A; Cattell, 1950).

2. *Disposition rigidity*—the neurotic has high perseveration scores on motor tests of perseveration (Himmelweit *et al.*, 1946; Eysenck, 1947; Cattell, 1950).

3. *Manual dexterity*—in a series of trials in a test of manual dexterity, the neurotic does not reach as high a score as the non-neurotic (Himmelweit *et al.*, 1946; Eysenck, 1947; Himmelweit and Petrie, 1951).

18

4. *Tempo of handwriting*—the neurotic writes more slowly (Himmelweit *et al.*, 1946; Eysenck, 1947).

5. *Self-rating*—the neurotic expresses greater inferiority feelings and self-criticism (Eysenck, 1947).

6. *Smoothness of work curve*—the neurotic has a more jagged work curve when a series of trials is given at a task (Himmelweit *et al.*, 1946; Eysenck, 1947).

The tests for each of these traits were chosen on the basis of their close relationship with the trait, and the convenience with which they could be used and scored.

Thus, for example, suggestibility is a generalised trait that manifests itself in various situations. The main feature in the tests which define this trait is the execution of a movement by any individual as a result of the repeated suggestion by the investigator that such a movement will take place without conscious participation in the movement of the subject. Among tests associated with this trait are:

(*a*) arm levitation, which involves raising the arm from the table when a strong suggestion is made;

(*b*) the Chevreul pendulum, in which the suggestion is made that a pendulum is swinging along a line which is drawn underneath it.

These tests are related to one another; that is, an individual who tends to behave in a certain way in one of these situations will behave in a similar way in the other. Of the various measures associated with this trait, the Body Sway Suggestibility test is most closely related and this is the test that we have used (Hull, 1933; Eysenck and Furneaux, 1945).[1]

CHANGES ON MEASUREMENTS RELATED TO 'NEUROTICISM' AFTER STANDARD LEUCOTOMY

Suggestibility

The Body Sway test of motor suggestibility used consisted basically of asking the patient to stand in a relaxed position with his eyes closed for two minutes whilst the suggestion is repeatedly made to him that he is falling forward. By means of

[1] This test has been shown to differentiate between the neurotic and the non-neurotic and has been found to discriminate between extreme neurotics and patients suffering from milder forms of the illness.

a thread—attached to the collar of the patient and ending in a weight swinging freely on a scale—the amount of sway during this period is measured. Three months after posterior Standard leucotomy there was a marked decrease in suggestibility as measured by the amount of sway. After nine months the decrease in suggestibility was still further accentuated.

Disposition Rigidity; Perseveration Tests

The patient carried out a task which necessitated his shifting from an habitual activity to a non-habitual one. He first wrote the figures 2, 3, 4 in the usual manner; he then wrote each starting from the base of the numeral instead of the top (Cattell, 1946B; Petrie, 1948A). The ratio of his output at the two tasks during the same time interval is his perseveration score. If his performance at the new task is poorer than that on the old, he has a high perseveration score. This particular test is one that is closely related to the general tendency towards rigidity in such situations. Three months after the operation the patient showed greater facility in shifting from the habitual task to the non-habitual task; that is, he had a lower perseveration score.

An additional test was used in which the alternation was between two tasks neither of which involved the creation of a new habit. A five-letter word was written in the usual manner; then the order of the letters was reversed. The patient also showed decreased rigidity on this second test, although it did not reach the level of significance. Thus three months after leucotomy the patient on two tests of perseveration showed a tendency to be more flexible in shifting from one kind of activity to another of related type.

Nine months after the operation the decrease in rigidity was maintained. Again a significant difference was found on the test which involved the alternation of a relatively new activity with an habitual one. There were lower perseveration scores in the alternation of two tasks which did not involve the formation of a new habit, but this was only a suggestive change.

Manual Dexterity

In order to arrive at the highest score on a series of trials on a test involving manual dexterity, each of the patients was given eight trials on the Track Tracer (a machine kindly loaned by

Professor Bartlett from the Cambridge Psychological Laboratory). On this test the patient has to trace with a metal stylus a winding path which runs between two rows of holes on an ivorine sheet. Each time the stylus touches a hole a connection is made with a metal plate underneath the ivorine cover, an electric counter is activated and a buzzer sounds (Himmelweit, 1946; Eysenck, 1947).

Three months after the operation the top score achieved during these eight trials was significantly greater than before; that is, on the 'best' trial the time in which the patients managed to complete the work was considerably less than before the operation. After nine months the 'best' trial of the eight was even more markedly improved.

Tempo of Handwriting

The speed of writing was measured by asking patients to write the word 'ready' as often as possible in one minute. Nine months after the operation the speed was significantly greater than before. (The increase in speed was not apparent at three months.)

Self-criticism

In order to arrive at a measure of self-criticism, a quantitative self-rating was obtained, the patients stating whether they thought they did or did not exhibit each of forty-two unpleasant traits often ascribed to himself by the neurotic. There was a decided decrease in the number of unpleasant traits ascribed to themselves after the operation. This decrease in self-criticism was shown at three months and again at nine months.

Smoothness of Work Curve

On two separate measures we found smoother work curves after three months. The first was the rate of tapping in four quarter-minute periods. The second was in the speed of completing the eight trials on the Track Tracer. It was found that the mean deviation from the average in tapping was greater before than after the operation. On the Track Tracer the number of 'relapses', that is, the losses in speed in the course of the trials, was greater prior to the operation than afterwards.

After nine months the smoother work curves were not so noticeable. We did find, however, that in one case the increase was significant in the right direction. This was the number of figures given in a series of eight trials of concentration (Appendix A—Test 14). There was a smoother curve in the speed of tapping in four quarter-minutes, but this was only suggestive.

DISCUSSION AND SUMMARY REGARDING NEUROTICISM

What is important in all this is that, in regard to six traits which are associated with neuroticism, we have obtained significant changes after leucotomy, all in the direction of a decrease in neuroticism; that is, the patient is less suggestible, shows less disposition rigidity, has a higher 'top score' in a series of trials on a test of manual dexterity, has a faster tempo in handwriting, exhibits less self-criticism and has smoother work curves. We found this after three months and again after nine months. The pattern of changes was as clearly shown after the short as after the longer period; only in the case of the smoothness of the work curves was it less pronounced after the longer period.

If the patient has changed in that he has moved away from the neurotic end of the dimension 'neuroticism', we would also expect to find changes in a definite direction on some of the other tests we used. In fact such changes were found, although they did not reach the level of significance. He swayed less when he was standing in a relaxed position and asked to close his eyes; higher scores on this test (Static Ataxia) are found in a neurotic population (Eysenck, 1947; Himmelweit and Petrie, 1951).

Wechsler (1944) reports that on his scale of intelligence tests neurotics and unstable individuals tend to do badly on the Digit Substitution test. He suggests that the poorer mental efficiency of the neurotic is displayed by his low performance in this test. Our patients improved on this test after the operation.[1]

These two suggestive changes lend further support to the conclusion we have come to on the basis of significant changes on six traits—that the patient after posterior Standard leucotomy showed a decrease in 'neuroticism'.

[1] See Chapter III.

22

CHANGE IN TEMPERAMENT

We have described earlier the identification of a dimension of personality, at one end of which is the extraverted individual and at the other the introverted individual. Certain traits have been shown to be associated with this dimension in a neurotic population.

The introvert patient in contrast to the extravert is characterised by:

1. A tendency to aim at accuracy rather than speed (Himmelweit, 1946; Eysenck, 1947; Petrie, 1948A; Cattell, 1950).

2. A tendency to self-blame rather than blame of the environment; that is, a tendency to intropunitiveness (Rosenzweig and Sarason, 1942; Hunt, 1944).

3. A preoccupation with the past rather than the present and future (Eysenck, 1947; Petrie, 1948A).

4. A low rating of sex humour (Eysenck, 1947; Cattell, 1950).

5. A high verbal score in relation to performance score on intelligence tests (Himmelweit, 1945; Eysenck, 1947; Cattell, 1950).

If the hypothesis of a decrease in introversion after leucotomy is correct we should expect to find changes on these traits in the direction of the extraverted end of the scale.

Speed and Accuracy

In view of both the theoretical and practical importance of changes in behaviour affecting speed and accuracy, it was decided to examine a number of different tasks involving both mental and manual activity.

Accuracy

The patients are more inaccurate three months after posterior Standard leucotomy. On a manual task, the Track Tracer, they made more mistakes after the operation, this being shown on the second and the penultimate trials in the series and the total number on all trials. On Porteus Mazes test, where the patient finds his way out of a series of ten mazes of increasing difficulty, more errors occurred after leucotomy.

There was also an increase in the number of mistakes made in producing as many words as possible out of the letters comprising a nine-letter word. The patient produced more words which are not to be found in any dictionary and more frequently repeated a word that had already been listed. The number of mistakes in the Arithmetic, Picture Completion and Picture Arrangement tests on the Wechsler scale had also increased. Thus increased inaccuracy is noticeable in mental as well as in manual tasks.

The changes after nine months indicate that the patients' tendency to make more mistakes is still present. There is even some evidence that it has been accentuated. Both on a manual task—the eight trials on the Track Tracer—and on the planning task—involving drawing a path out of a series of ten mazes—more mistakes occurred. The number of errors in mental tasks also shows a further increase at nine months. This was exemplified in the mistakes on the Arithmetic, the Picture Arrangement and Picture Completion tests of the Wechsler. There is thus a distinct tendency for patients after leucotomy to be more inaccurate in many different types of work.

Speed

In addition to the increase in the number of mistakes made on the mazes and the Track Tracer which we have mentioned above, these tasks were carried out more quickly three months after leucotomy. Furthermore, the speed in the Arithmetic and the Picture Arrangement tests on the Wechsler scale had increased. Thus there is an increase in the speed of completing primarily mental tasks as well as manual tasks.

Nine months after the operation there was ample evidence that the patients' tendency to be quicker was still present; and some evidence that they were quicker than three months after leucotomy. On the manual task, the eight trials on the Track Tracer, they worked at greater speed. They also completed the ten Porteus mazes in less time. This decrease in time on the mazes is particularly striking, as if a mistake is made it is necessary to do the whole maze again. This involves going back to the beginning and 'wasting' again the time it has taken to arrive at the site of the mistake.

The speed of mental tasks maintains its increase; thus the

24

speed of decision in rating pictorial humour had increased suggestively and on the Arithmetic and Picture Arrangement of the Wechsler test is greater. Hence after nine months the patients, in both mental and manual tasks, show the same tendency as they did at the earlier investigation; they tackle the job more quickly.

These various findings indicate a distinct tendency for the patients after leucotomy to have a preference for speed rather than accuracy. It is difficult to say whether the increase in the number of mistakes they make is related to their doing things at a greater speed, although these two variables have been shown to be related on the Track Tracer (Himmelweit, 1946). We tried to obtain some evidence regarding this in leucotomy patients by examining the increase in speed which accompanied errors on two tests. The time taken over the questions on which a failure had been made after, but not before, leucotomy was compared with those in which the correct answer had been given on both occasions on the Arithmetic and Picture Arrangement tests of the Wechsler. It was found that the speed had increased on both 'failed' and 'non-failed' questions, though more conspicuously on the 'failed' questions. We have therefore no conclusive evidence to show that the mistakes are due to the speed preference.

Many writers who have observed this tendency in leucotomy patients have described it in their clinical interpretations as an increase in impulsiveness; others have described a decrease in cautiousness. It is partly a question of taste whether one phrase is preferred to the other, the facts are as stated; the patients are quicker and make many more mistakes in both mental and manual tasks after the operation.

It would seem desirable in weighing up the advantages and disadvantages of operating in the case of neurotics to bear the occupational factor in mind and the effect on their efficiency of this expected change of temperament. There is every reason to believe that this finding on so many different tasks, all present both after three months and the longer period, will display itself in the day-to-day life of the patient. Two examples given by Tiffin (1946) about normal industrial workers are relevant. In the inspection of tin plates it was found that the number of defects noted did not increase even when four times as much time was spent. On the other hand, in such a task as punch pressing, an increased speed is disadvantageous because the nature of the task is such that the number of mistakes made is closely related to the speed at which it is performed—the greater the speed, the greater the number of mistakes.

Reaction to Frustration

It has been shown that stress in the face of obstacles produces different types of reaction which can be grouped in a threefold division (Rosenzweig, 1938). Responses in which the individual attributes the frustration to external persons or things are called 'extrapunitive'; responses in which the individual aggressively attributes the frustration to himself are called 'intropunitive'. A third type of response, when an attempt is made to avoid blame altogether, whether of others or of oneself, and to gloss over the frustrating situation, is called 'impunitive'. It has been shown that a very high incidence of the intropunitive type of response is found in the introverted group of neurotics (Rosenzweig, 1944). These intropunitive responses are associated with emotions of guilt and remorse.

It was decided to examine the effect of leucotomy on the patients' reaction to two types of stress. Firstly, internal stress, in the form of his own incapacities of character; secondly, external stress, in the form of an insoluble problem.

Tendency towards Self-blame

Intropunitive reactions to personal incapacities

As an estimate of the tendency towards self-blame it had been arranged for patients to state whether or not they considered that they were characterised by forty-two unpleasant traits; they then stated whether they blamed themselves for any of these traits. For example, if they regarded themselves as being cowardly, they stated whether they blamed themselves for the cowardice. By using a three-point scale we were able to obtain some indication of the intensity of the self-blame they experienced as a result of their failings.

Three months after leucotomy the patients' attitude towards themselves had changed. They blamed themselves for significantly fewer characteristics. Moreover, where there was still a feeling of blame it was less intense. After nine months still fewer of the unpleasant characteristics are regarded as blame-worthy, and where there is blame it tends to be little rather than very much.

Traits which had caused some of the patients to torture them-selves with guilt feelings prior to the operation appeared to be relatively unimportant afterwards. They may still regard them-selves, for example, as being moody or irritable, but they accept the fact; it does not induce guilt feelings to the same extent nor of the same intensity. As one of the patients said, 'I know I am moody but, after all, that is me, like the colour of my eyes.' This will mean probably that the leucotomy patient will be less pre-occupied with improving himself; he will feel there is less to improve and that improvement is not very important. But he will be a happier person as a result and to this extent, at any rate, may be a source of happiness to the people round him.

This change was demonstrated rather dramatically in one patient, a housewife of the lower middle class. Prior to her operation there was hardly a single unpleasant personality trait which she did not regard herself as possessing. She was riddled with guilt feelings and as a result was all but unbearable to her family. Afterwards her husband stated that living with her had never been so pleasant as it was now when, in talking of her characteristics, she gave the impression of describing a different person.

Reaction to external frustration: an insoluble task

The marked decrease in self-blame found in patients after leucotomy had raised the question as to where their blame was directed. The general impression gained from the patients' account of their characteristics after the operation was that they tended increasingly to feel that the responsibility for their irritability or their extravagance lay in the world round them, as opposed to themselves.

At the end of the series of Porteus mazes, each patient was presented with an insoluble maze and was told that he would be given half a minute to try and complete it. This period was not long enough for the patient to realise that there was, in fact, no way out of this particular maze. At the end of the half-minute the maze was taken away and the patient was asked,

'You know I am interested in what *you* think. I have asked you many questions to-day about your own attitudes and beliefs. Please tell me now why you think you could not do that maze?' The patients' answers were noted down verbatim.

Our hypothesis was that after the operation patients would show decreased intropunitiveness; that is, they would provide fewer explanations related to their own inadequacy, their own psychological traits, and would tend increasingly to consider the nature of the problem, or the conditions surrounding it, responsible for their failures. But in order to make certain that these were not subjective interpretations based on the hypothesis with which we had planned this investigation, the answers were independently analysed by two other psychologists, Dr. Johanna Krout of the Psychological Institute, Chicago, and Miss Maryse Israel, Lecturer in Psychology at the Institute of Psychiatry, London University, to both of whom I am greatly indebted for their help on this and other aspects of the work.

For this analysis the answers given before and after leucotomy were rearranged in random order, so that the individual evaluating them did not know whether these particular explanations were given before or after the operation. The three judges agreed about the general trend, and these trends supported the hypothesis on which we had originally planned this investigation. Thus, before the operation there were many more answers such as 'I am too slow'; 'I don't try enough'; 'I am not that brilliant'; 'I am over-anxious'; and 'lack of concentration'. After the operation there were many more explanations such as 'this problem is too complex'; 'it has too many lines'; 'there are too many openings'; 'it cannot be done in the time'; and so on. This change, when considered in terms of the percentage of answers blaming failure on to the nature of the problem instead of their own inadequacy, reached the level of significance; it was present at three months and was even more definite at nine months.

It is clear that in the everyday life of the patient, which will not be free of frustrating situations, this difference in reaction and outlook will have considerable repercussions on behaviour and happiness. The tendency 'to blame the tools' manifested itself also during many of the situations in the hours we spent with the patients. It was noticed very often after the operation that inability to complete a task was accompanied by a remark which suggested that patients believed the task could not be done. For example, in doing the jigsaw puzzles of the Wechsler scale the patients would say, 'Aren't there some pieces missing here?' Or during one of the earlier mazes which are soluble, they would suggest that there was no way out.

Thus, from two separate approaches, there is evidence, using Rosenzweig's terminology, of a decrease in intropunitiveness; and we have also been able to obtain objective evidence of blame being directed to the environment instead of to the self.

Attitude to Time

Israeli's (1936) investigation into attitude to time led him to conclude that an examination of the patient's outlook on the past and future is a salient approach to understanding that individual. The subjective attitude to the past, present and future of patients before and after Standard posterior leucotomy was obtained from their answers to eight standardised questions based on Israeli's (1936) work. These questions and answers were given verbally and were presented in the form, 'Which do you think about most—(a) the past, (b) the present or (c) the future?'

The questions were as follows:

1. Which do you think about most, a, b or c?
2. Which do you think about least?
3. Which do you feel least unhappy about?
4. Which do you feel most unhappy about?
5. Which do you worry about most?
6. Which do you worry about least?
7. Which are you most interested in?
8. Which are you least interested in?

Three months after leucotomy, in answering Question 4, 36% of the patients had ceased being most unhappy about the present; on Question 5, 26% of the patients had ceased finding the present their main cause of worry; and on Question 3, 23% had ceased being most happy about the past. After nine months more pronounced changes in the same direction occurred in these three answers: on Question 4, 51%; on Question 5, 25%; and on Question 3, 43% respectively.

Three months after leucotomy there was an increase of 43% in those who were most unhappy about the past (Question 4a), an increase of 16% in those least interested in the past (Question 8a), and an increase of 11% in those who had become least unhappy about the present (Question 3b). A more pronounced change occurred in the same direction at nine months; the percentages were 43% (Question 4a), 24% (Question 8a) and 23% (Question 3b) respectively.

There was also an interesting change in attitudes towards the future. At three months there was an increase of 22% in those who were most happy about the future (Question 3c), and 11% who were most happy about the present (Question 3b). At nine months there was an increase of 25% on those who were most happy about the future (Question 3c) and an increase of 23% in those who were most happy about the present (Question 3b). Although not reaching the level of significance, there is an increase after the operation in those who think least about the future. This is in agreement with the comments that have been made suggesting that after leucotomy patients tend to live predominantly in the present.

Thus, after leucotomy we have a picture of an individual who is much more absorbed by, and lives much more happily in, the present than he did before his operation, who tends to leave the past behind him and who, when he does consider the future, is more reassured. This is in contrast with his state of mind before the operation, which tended to be oriented towards the past and was highly dissatisfied with the present. The picture is reasonably clear at three months. After the further interval there is an accentuation of the tendency to 'let the dead past bury its dead', and contentment with the present—it would seem almost at the expense of the future.

Appreciation of Sex Humour

To measure changes in the appreciation of humour after leucotomy the patient was given a series of twenty-five pictorial jokes which had been collected from various magazines. These included jokes which were primarily concerned with sex and also 'neutral' jokes which had no obvious relation to sex. The patient was asked to decide about each joke, whether he considered it to be 'extremely amusing', 'amusing', 'slightly amusing' or 'not amusing'. He was allowed to take as long as he wished to decide into which of these categories to place it.

Three months after the operation some of the jokes 'moved up' in rating; that is, the group of patients taken as a whole tended to find certain jokes 'extremely amusing' which previous to the operation had been rated 'slightly amusing' or 'amusing'; or a joke that had been 'not amusing' became one that was 'amusing'.

The jokes that 'moved up' the scale were examined. It was found that they were all of the type in which the humour hinged on the sexual content; that is, no 'neutral' jokes were found by the group as a whole to be more amusing after the operation.

After nine months the rating of the jokes gave an even clearer impression of the patients' tendency to be more amused by sex jokes.

The jokes that went up the scale at this third investigation were, as a psychiatrist asked to describe them said, 'pure pornography'. No 'neutral' joke went up in value. Moreover, in the case of some of the patients, a number of the sex jokes changed in rating from being 'slightly amusing' to being 'extremely amusing', skipping a category on their way up the scale; changes of this extent did not occur with any of the 'neutral' jokes.

An example of the 'neutral' type of joke that did *not* go up in value was picture No. 1.

An example of the sex joke that did go up in value was picture No. 2.

Differential Loss on Verbal and Performance Intelligence

The patients were given four verbal tests and four performance tests of the Wechsler scale of intelligence. This provided a verbal I.Q. and a performance I.Q.[1] Three months after leucotomy they had lost on verbal intelligence test scores, but

[1] The Wechsler Verbal tests were the Comprehension, Similarities, Digits, and Arithmetic. The Wechsler Performance tests were the Picture Arrangement, Picture Completion, Object Assembly and Digit Symbol.

The Vocabulary test was also used, but in order to retain the balance between the Verbal and Performance Sections of the scale, this score was not included in estimating the I.Q.

not on performance test scores (see Chapter III). After nine months this differential loss persisted; the patient showed a significant loss on verbal I.Q. and a slight insignificant gain on performance I.Q. Thus the patient after leucotomy had a higher performance score in relation to his verbal score than prior to leucotomy.

These changes on intellectual measurements might be regarded as being partly due to the alteration in temperament. The post-leucotomy patient is quicker and more inaccurate, so that he gains on intelligence tests—such as those in the performance scale—where extra points are earned for speed; and loses on tests where speed is no advantage and impulsiveness is even penalised, as on some of the verbal tests.

If this differential loss is partly due to the effect of a temperamental change, it might throw some light on the causes of the difference in intelligence scores amongst extraverts and introverts. It had been thought that introverts tended to be preoccupied with reading and associated interests and developed as a result a facility for dealing with problems involving words (Himmelweit, 1945). It may be that differences in speed and accuracy, for example, are affecting their intelligence score.

It is of interest that one of the clinicians has pointed out that a high ratio of verbal to performance test scores is prognostically of value in deciding upon leucotomy when clinical signs are indefinite (Frank, 1946).[1]

Endurance

A number of situations involving endurance in an uncomfortable physical position have been shown to be related to one another (Ryans, 1939; Himmelweit and Petrie, 1951). For example, the length of time grip can be maintained on a dynamometer—at half the maximum—is closely related to the length of time the leg can be held without support, or the time that the same individual can remain standing on tiptoe. It has been shown that such tests are a good indication of an

---

[1] An individual who has low verbal intelligence in comparison with performance intelligence may not be able to afford the loss on verbal intelligence which will result from his operation; this, therefore, might constitute an indication against leucotomy. Details of an investigation to determine objective prognostic indicators are presented in Chapter V.

individual's capacity of endurance in normal life (Ryans, 1939; Cureton et al., 1945). There is also evidence that these measurements of endurance are an indication of the tendency or otherwise of an individual to work towards the point of complete exhaustion (Jones, 1948). Thus, apart from the difference in behaviour of introverts and extraverts on such tests (Eysenck, 1947; Petrie, 1948A) they would appear to be a measure of a socially important trait.

The test of endurance we used was the 'leg test', in which the patient is asked to hold up the leg in an uncomfortable position as long as possible. Three months after leucotomy the patient gave up earlier at this task. After nine months the diminution in endurance is still more marked. This might be because he became tired more quickly than before the operation or that he gave way to tiredness more quickly. Whichever is the explanation, a marked loss in endurance was found.[1]

DISCUSSION AND SUMMARY REGARDING INTROVERSION

In tests of the six traits related to the dimension extraversion-introversion there was a change in the direction of a decrease in introversion. The patient was more inaccurate and worked at greater speed; showed a diminished tendency to blame himself; was less oriented towards the past than to the present and future; liked sex humour better. The ratio of verbal to performance intelligence score dropped and he showed less physical endurance. This pattern of change was clearly shown three months and nine months after Standard posterior leucotomy; in some cases it was accentuated after the longer period (Petrie, 1949A and B).

If the patient has changed in so far as he has moved away from the introverted end of the scale, we would expect to find a change on another test which we used—that of Level of Aspiration.

To arrive at a measure of the patient's goal-setting behaviour, a series of trials were given on the Track Tracer which has already been described. The patient was asked, after a practice

[1] It has been decided to consider tests of physical endurance separately from tests of persistence at a task because there is some indication in the literature that although they are positively correlated and both are related to neuroticism, tests of endurance are specially related to the introvert-extravert dimension (Eysenck, 1947; Petrie, 1948A).

trial, to judge how good his previous trial had been and to state what his goal was going to be for the coming trial. Eight trials were given and the total of these judgments and goals was used in arriving at our results.

The Track Tracer is designed so that the mistakes are counted on an electric counter and a bell rings when a mistake is made. Goal and judgment were measured both in terms of the time taken, or to be taken, and the number of mistakes made, or to be made.

Changes were found in this test but they did not reach the level of significance. There was a tendency for the patients to set themselves lower goals after the operation. There was also a tendency in some of the scores for capacity to be over-estimated. Perhaps because of the other temperament changes found after leucotomy this pattern, however, was not clearly shown. It has been reported that after the operation there was an increase in the number of mistakes made and in the speed of working on the Track Tracer. There was some evidence to suggest that this change was so great as to hide the alteration in the pattern of goal-setting behaviour with regard to speed and accuracy. On the first two trials in which the patient's estimate of goal was obtained he was unaware of his actual performance; that is, he set himself a 'blind' goal based on a 'blind' estimation. On these 'blind' trials it was noted that the patient's goal dropped in comparison with his pre-operative behaviour both with regard to time and mistakes, at three months and nine months after the operation. It seems likely that if the other variables could be omitted, one would obtain a clear pattern of the lowering of goals. It would thus appear advisable to measure the level of aspiration in leucotomy patients on a test which does not involve speed and accuracy or any of the other traits on which they show considerable changes.

Diminished introversion would also lead us to expect a change in attitude to pictorial humour, as it has been shown that extraverts tend to appreciate all types of humour more than do introverts (Eysenck, 1947). A change in attitude to pictorial humour of various types was found but it did not reach the level of significance.

It was mentioned earlier on that we had given the patients twenty-five jokes which were to be rated 'extremely amusing', 'slightly amusing', 'amusing' or 'not amusing'. There was one finding suggestive of a general tendency to appreciate pictorial humour more after the operation: this was that fewer jokes were placed in the category 'not amusing' after the operation than before the operation. Most of the items which had previously been recorded as 'not amusing' were regarded after the operation as 'slightly amusing'. This is not the sort of change which one would expect to find when individuals are presented for the second time with a number of jokes. For example, Cattell and Luborsky (1947) report an experiment in which jokes were readministered after five months to one hundred subjects of both sexes. At the second administration a lowering of humour scores was found. Leucotomy patients find more jokes amusing even when presented with the same set of jokes for the third time.[1]

Thus, in addition to significant changes on six traits associated with diminished introversion, we have found other suggestive test changes in the same direction present three months and nine months after the operation. In combination they lend support to the hypothesis that posterior Standard leucotomy results in diminished introversion.

In addition to the changes in personality which we have attempted to measure objectively, there are two other general characteristics of extraverts which remind us of our post-leucotomy population. Among such general characteristics are the extraverts' own reports that they are 'accident prone' (Eysenck, 1947). We have reported in detail the many directions from which evidence has been obtained of the great speed at which patients tackle a task after leucotomy, and the accompanying large number of errors in their activity. This was shown in manual tasks as well as mental tasks. Making a large number of mistakes in a manual task—on an assembly line, driving a motor car or looking after the running of any other machine—does in fact lead to their being more liable to suffer accidents. This suggests an increase in leucotomy patients of a

[1] The shift in humour rating is possibly also indicative of alteration in enthusiasm. The change from the 'not amusing' category to the 'slightly amusing' category may be an indication of the increased 'neutral' attitude of patients after leucotomy, an absence of both strong negative and positive feelings—in fact, an attitude which finds 'slightly amusing' the most favoured category.

characteristic ascribed to themselves by extraverts. The patients' behaviour suggests that they would, after the operation, be more 'accident prone'.

There is another point which differentiates the patient after leucotomy from his preleucotomy state which is reminiscent of the difference between the introvert and the extravert, although the cause of this difference is unlikely to be the same in the two populations. The post-leucotomy patient tends to be fatter than the preleucotomy patient. The extravert has been shown to have greater girth in relation to height, whilst the introvert has greater height in relation to girth (Rees and Eysenck, 1945; Rees, 1950). The explanation of this difference is so complex that it will not be further pursued, but it does pose the question as to whether a different temperament in extraverts might be a factor in determining a difference in physique.

MISCELLANEOUS TESTS

Previous investigations have suggested that the patients were more distractible after leucotomy (Freeman and Watts, 1942; Frankl and Mayer-Gross, 1947; and Partridge, 1950); that they had decreased in fluency (Rylander, 1948); and there were many reports of a change in attitude towards their illness.

Concentration and Distractibility

In the test of concentration we used, the patient was asked to repeat groups of figures from a series which was interrupted at irregular intervals. At three months there was a slight insignificant decrease in scores, indicating somewhat greater difficulty in concentrating. At nine months this tendency was reversed; the patients had higher scores on this test of concentration, although the improvement is not statistically significant.

A test of distractibility was devised which involved doing the same task as was required in the Concentration test, namely, repeating groups of figures from a series which was interrupted at irregular intervals—but the reading of the figures was accompanied by the ringing of a raucous telephone bell. Distractibility was measured by the difference between concentration with and without the distraction of the telephone bell.

At three months the patients appeared to be less distractible than before the operation. At nine months this finding was reversed. There was a suggestive increase in distractibility. (It will be remembered that at three months the patients were also concentrating less well than before the operation; this may have hidden the tendency to increased distractibility that appeared after the longer period.)

On the Concentration test there is another finding which hints at improvement. There is a suggestion of a more consistent level of ability as there is less variation in number of digits remembered during the eight trials; that is, prior to leucotomy a patient would in the series of trials remember five figures, then only one figure, then two. After leucotomy there was a tendency to remember always four or always three. This was not the case in the Distractibility test, on which the patient had poorer scores after leucotomy and no suggestion of a more consistent level of performance.

The finding suggestive of improved concentration is in line with the report in the Greystone Project (Mettler, 1949), where no impairment of immediate memory was found, and in some cases an improvement was noted. Other findings in this project, such as an increase in recognition ability after the operation, also suggest greater ability to concentrate. This change may, however, be associated with the decrease in emotional conflict —the fewer 'internal distractions'—rather than with an absolute increase in the ability to concentrate.

Fluctuation or Reversal of Perspective

The fluctuations in an ambiguous figure are a cause of one of the difficulties in trying to teach solid geometry on a blackboard. Unless solid objects are drawn with such shading that they can be seen in one way only, the alternate interpretation continues to present itself. Thus, a corridor drawn without any shading can be seen as going away from you or jutting out towards you and the two interpretations tend to alternate. The rate of fluctuations of an ambiguous figure is reported to be related to other aspects of personality (McDougall, 1926; Cattell, 1950).

We used Necker's Cube in order to measure the number of reversals of perspective occurring during a period of a minute. The patient was asked first to let it reverse and not to try and speed it up or slow it down. During a further period of a minute

37

he was asked to try and make the cube change as often as possible.

After leucotomy, at the three months' retest, the number of fluctuations on an ambiguous figure in a period of a minute had suggestively increased. This change reached the level of significance when the patient attempted to increase the number of fluctuations; that is, when his will was consciously being exercised. The difference, moreover, between 'willed' and 'unwilled' fluctuations had increased after the operation and was significant both at three months and at nine months. This finding—indicative of more effective control in this situation—is in line with the decreased suggestibility reported earlier in this chapter and with other results suggesting that in tasks involving control, such as concentration and perseveration, the patient may have a better performance after leucotomy. This leaves open the question of whether the patient's will is stronger or whether it has less to contend with in the way of conflicting impulses.

An associated alteration in mental imagery is suggested by the findings of Gordon (1950). She examined the relationship between the rate of fluctuation and mental imagery and found that the control of fluctuation—as measured in this investigation (reported in Appendix A, Test 15)—was significantly related to less vivid and controlled imagery. Suggestion of a loss in vividness of imagery after leucotomy was also found in the spontaneous essays which the patients wrote. Additional evidence of this comes from Crown's (1951) work on the interpretation of Rorschach Ink Blots with psychotics who have undergone leucotomy. It may be that the patient after leucotomy can control his imagery better, but this may ensue from a lesser vitality in his imagery.

An attempt might be made to explain the increased control of fluctuation as a measure of the greater co-operativeness of post-leucotomy patients. It might be suggested that they may be more motivated to do what the examiner asks. This explanation, however, is not borne out by the behaviour of patients on other tests. For example, in the endurance test the patient was asked to hold his leg up as long as possible. If he was more co-operative after the operation it might have been expected that he would hold the leg up longer; in fact he maintained this position for a considerably shorter time, as was reported earlier in this chapter. The second example is on the Track Tracer; asked to make as few mistakes as possible, he made more after the operation.

Time Judgment

A duration of time judgment investigation was incorporated because of the possibility that there might be a change in this which would throw light on the reported loss of foresight and the tendency to work at greater speed which has been found in so many different tasks.

In our experiment we obtained a judgment of both unfilled and filled time; that is, when the patient was doing nothing and when he was occupied. In the former he reproduced the time intervals; in the latter he made a verbal estimate of a period of time.

The judgment of unfilled time was made for a 15-second and a 60-second period: 15 seconds was measured on a stopwatch and an indication was given when this had passed; the patient then made his own estimate of 15 seconds. The same procedure was repeated for a period of 60 seconds. (He was requested to refrain from counting 'in his mind' during both parts of the test.)

The filled time period was the length of time he thought he took to complete the second trial on the Track Tracer. This was always longer than 30 seconds and less than one and a half minutes.

Both at three months and nine months—both for filled and unfilled time—the patient reported time as going more quickly, although when considered individually these changes were not completely significant. He thought a minute had passed more quickly than previous to his operation, and he thought that the time he had taken over his trial on the Track Tracer was longer than previously. Thus there is a suggestion in the results that time seems to be passing more quickly after leucotomy.

Fluency

When we have found a change in a personality trait which is statistically significant three months after Standard leucotomy, and have confirmed its presence nine months after, we can be reasonably certain that when the operation is performed on this type of patient such a change will occur. But if we have failed to find a change of a certain trait we cannot be equally certain that it is not present. It is possible that the test was faulty, or that the alteration was too small to show significantly in a population of this size.

But one of the negative findings in this investigation does appear to be worth reporting. This was on the two Fluency tests used. The present writer (Petrie, 1948A) had investigated the closeness of relationship between various Fluency tests in a neurotic population. A general trait of fluency was found and the two tests used in this investigation were closely related to this trait. These were:

1. The number of round objects that could be named in the period of a minute (Cattell, 1936).
2. The number of objects that could be suggested for insertion into a picture of a tree (Cattell, 1936).

Three months after the operation we found a slight insignificant loss on these tests. This was reversed at the longer period when a gain was found, though it did not reach the level of significance. The slight loss found at three months is in line with Crown's (1951) results in his interesting investigation of the effects of leucotomy on a psychotic population. He followed up each case at three months and found a loss in fluency. On the other hand, our finding of a gain at nine months is at variance with Rylander (1948), who has done a follow-up on his psychotic patients after a longer period and reports a loss in fluency. The discrepancy between Rylander's findings and those reported in this book may be due to the type of population, the type of operation and type of test. Rylander carried out investigations on a psychotic population; and the operation performed by the neurosurgeon in Sweden is different from that which is used by McKissock (1943). Moreover, Rylander used as his measure of fluency the number of nouns that could be mentioned in a given time. Fruchter (1948) has demonstrated that verbal fluency is made up of several factors, one of which is called 'single word fluency'. This is probably what Rylander is measuring. We, on the other hand, have been using tests which are better grouped under Fruchter's second fluency factor of 'controlled association'.

Thus, although it has not reached the level of significance, our findings tend to suggest that if there is a change in fluency in this kind of population following on leucotomy, it shows itself as a gain after the longer interval and not a loss such as has been suggested by the two workers mentioned above.

Traits on which Patients regard themselves as changed

We previously referred to a list of forty-two unpleasant traits frequently ascribed to themselves by neurotics. It was reported that the patients tended to ascribe fewer unpleasant traits to themselves after leucotomy. An attempt was made to ascertain on which traits the patient regarded himself as having changed by comparing each of these forty-two items for each of the patients before and nine months after the operation. The most pronounced differences were found with regard to the questions 'Are you despondent?' and 'Are you fussy?' 58% of the patients had ceased to regard themselves as being despondent and 42% ceased to regard themselves as fussy.

Significant changes were also found in the following: patients had ceased to consider themselves as silly, selfish, naggers, unco-operative, hostile, resentful, hesitant, unconscientious and bad-tempered.

It is not suggested that this is an accurate objective description of the post-leucotomy patient, but this is how the patient after leucotomy regards himself. It is a self-portrait of an individual not over-blessed with insight who tends, as we have shown, to over-rate himself and to have lower standards than prior to his operation.

In this setting it is of interest to note the traits on which the group of patients as a whole did *not* regard themselves as having improved; that is, the traits which they ascribed to themselves both before and after the operation. They continued to regard themselves as being lazy, moody, careless and uninterested in people. Moreover, two traits were more frequently ascribed to themselves after the operation than before, although this change did not reach the level of significance. The group as a whole tended to regard itself as more irritable and more extravagant. It may be that we have here an indication of the undesirable traits reported by the family and friends of the patient.

This self-portrait, therefore, presents an individual who is much more satisfied with his buoyancy and his ability to leave people and things alone; and who appears to have some inkling that he may be extravagant and that he may be momentarily more put out by unpleasant circumstances. As many of these patients prior to the operation suffered greatly as a result of subjective attitudes, the alteration in viewing their own personality is by no means irrelevant to the improvement following on leucotomy.

Attitude to Illness

Prefrontal leucotomy is intended to relieve the illness of the individual operated upon.   In a psychotic population it is less common for a patient to realise that he is ill. In a neurotic population, such as that which forms the basis of this investigation, the individual often has sufficient insight to realise that he is ill.

Sixteen (80%) of our patients stated prior to the operation that they believed themselves to be ill. Seven (35%), moreover, thought that they would never get better. When one considers that this operation has the reputation of accomplishing that which is impossible by any other form of psychiatric treatment, the percentage of those who believed that they would not get better is a fairly good indication of their subjective hopelessness; so that we had here a population, a considerable proportion of whom, besides being troubled by their illness, were without hope that there would be any improvement in their health.

Three months after the operation only five (25%) of the patients considered themselves to be ill, and all of these believed that they would get better. The patients included in the investigation at nine months continued to show this striking change in their subjective attitude towards their illness. Six (30%) considered themselves to be ill and all but one of these believed they would get better. Thus, in addition to the clinical estimate of their better mental health, there is a noticeable improvement in their subjective beliefs about their condition. The change, perhaps particularly in those patients who prior to the operation were hopeless about any possibility of improvement, is indicative of a great reduction in human suffering.

CHAPTER III

THE EFFECT OF POSTERIOR STANDARD
LEUCOTOMY ON INTELLECTUAL ASPECTS
OF PERSONALITY

I N this chapter reports are presented of the changes found
after posterior Standard leucotomy on tests of intelligence,
and also changes in the style of writing and in the use of
language in speech.

In addition to the formal standardised tests of intelligence—
the Wechsler scale of verbal and performance tests, Porteus
Mazes and the proverbs from the Stanford Binet scale of intelligence—it was thought desirable to obtain from each patient
some written essays. It was hoped that if the patient was given
an opportunity to write about his friends and himself in his own
time, it might throw some light on the changes in temperament,
character and intelligence we found on other tests.

An alteration in the use of language was shown during the
administration of various tests and the definition of words
during a vocabulary test.

The patients were those described in Chapter II. They were
all tested on three occasions. The changes on twenty patients
found three months after the operation and nine months afterwards will be described. As with personality test results outlined
in the previous chapter, those differences which are statistically significant are reported as changes; that is, differences
which would occur by chance less than once in twenty (using
Fisher's 't' test). Statistical details will be found in Appendix B.

VARIETY OF INTELLECTUAL TESTS USED

It was decided to use a wide variety of intellectual tests. This
decision was based on the knowledge acquired in recent years of
the various separate facets of intelligence. It was possible that

after Standard posterior leucotomy intelligence might be affected in one aspect and not in another. An overall test of intelligence, therefore, might not show all the changes which had occurred, as loss in some aspects might be counterbalanced by gains in others. Moreover, inasmuch as temperament and character have been altered as a result of the operation, it was probable that there would be a different approach to certain types of tests but not to others.

These suppositions have proved to be correct and a loss was found only in certain aspects of intelligence.

Wechsler Bellevue Scale of Intelligence: Verbal and Performance Tests

As an adult population was being investigated, one of the tests we decided upon was the Wechsler Bellevue scale (1946), Form II, which was designed for the measurement of the intelligence of adults. This test was particularly suitable, as it samples a wide variety of intellectual activities and has been shown to be closely related to the practical correlates of intelligence, such as the degree of educational success. It assesses the individual's intelligence over a variety of tasks in terms of speed, quality and amount of production. One of its advantages is that the individual sub-tests can be separately analysed and give information about the specific function they are designed to measure.

It was decided that the advantages of using two different scales before and after leucotomy would be outweighed by the disadvantages. The Wechsler Form I scale has been shown to correlate with Form II scale only in so far as the total I.Q. scores are concerned; the individual sub-test shows low correlations (Gibby, 1950). Thus the identification of changes in the sub-tests would not have been possible had the two different forms been used.

The Wechsler test consists of a verbal scale and a performance scale. We used four verbal tests and four performance tests to arrive at the intelligence quotients. On the verbal side these were tests of social comprehension involving the description of appropriate behaviour in certain situations and the understanding of the reasons for a particular kind of behaviour in others; memory span—that is, the number of digits that can be retained and the number that can be reproduced in reverse order; the eduction of similarities—that is, the realisation of what is the element common to two objects; and mental arithmetic. On the performance side, the tests involved the identifying of missing portions of pictures; arranging drawings in an order which produces a sensible story; completing jigsaw puzzles; and a routine writing task involving the use of code.

In addition we gave a test of vocabulary requiring the definition of forty-five words; in order to retain the same number of verbal and performance tests, the score on the vocabulary test has not been included in the estimation of the intelligence quotients.

The usual results with individuals who are given these tests on two occasions is that they show improvement on the second application. Hamister (1949) and Derner *et al.* (1950), for example, found such improvement on retesting neurotic people after one week or one month.

We found that, three months after Standard posterior leucotomy, patients showed a loss on the verbal scale in contrast to the performance scale. The total loss on the four verbal tests was highly significant, whilst that on the four performance tests, though present, fell far short of the level of significance. Thus patients showed a loss in that aspect of intelligence which involved the use of words. This differential loss in verbal ability and performance ability is in agreement with the findings in other investigations (Crown, 1951).

In examining the four tests comprising the verbal scale it was found that only on one was the loss significant when taken alone. This was the Comprehension test, which consists of ten questions.

It was found that when each question was taken separately the loss was obvious on some of them but not on others. A list of the questions on which the loss was most pronounced was prepared. This list was then presented independently to three psychiatrists, who were asked to suggest what characterised the group of questions. There was considerable agreement between these three judges that the loss was most clearly shown on those questions eliciting social attitudes unrelated to the immediate environment.

Nine months after leucotomy the pattern of changes on the Wechsler test was essentially the same. There was a significant loss on the verbal scale—an average loss of 7 I.Q. points—and none on the performance scale. Indeed, there was a slight, though insignificant, gain in performance I.Q.

At the same time it was found that of the four verbal tests the loss on the Comprehension sub-test was significant when considered by itself, but that this was not the case with the remaining three tests.

An analysis of the answers to the ten questions making up the Comprehension test showed that patients nine months after Standard posterior leucotomy had significant loss on five of them. These five included enquiries regarding behaviour to prevent a train accident, the advantages of giving money to an organised charity rather than a street beggar, the reasons for using examinations to help in choosing civil servants and the reasons why a promise should be kept.

On the other hand, on a factual question, No. 9, asking for the reasons why cotton is suitable in making cloth, there was a slight, though non-significant, improvement.[1]

Thus the loss after the longer period also appears to be greatest on those questions requiring a patient to use social concepts unconnected with his immediate environment. This appears to suggest not only a loss in intellectual ability but a change in attitude towards the social environment. This impression is strengthened by the essays which each patient

[1] The Comprehension sub-test consists of ten questions. Those showing a significant loss at nine months are marked thus (−); a gain (insignificant) is marked thus (+).

	1.	What is the thing to do if you lose a book belonging to the library?
	2.	Why is it better to build a house with brick than of wood?
(−)	3.	What should you do if you see a train approaching a broken track?
(−)	4.	Why is it generally better to give money to an organised charity than to a street beggar?
	5.	What is the thing to do if a very good friend asks you for something you don't have?
	6.	Why are criminals locked up or put in prison?
(−)	7.	Why should most Government positions be filled through Civil Service Examinations?
(−)	8.	Why does the British Government require that a person wait from the time he makes application until the time he receives his final citizenship papers?
(+)	9.	Why is cotton used in making cloth?
(−)	10.	Why should a promise be kept?

produced describing a liked and a disliked individual, and himself as seen by these two people. After the operation, social qualities connected with relationship to society at large were less frequently mentioned in the four essays. This and other findings will be reported in greater detail in the relevant section at the end of this chapter.

Wechsler (1944) suggests that one might describe the Comprehension test as being a test of 'commonsense'. He stated that it includes a certain amount of practical information and a general ability to evaluate past experience. If this is the case it would appear that our patients have not lost so much on the amount of practical information at their disposal; they have changed, according to Wechsler's terminology, in their evaluation of past experience.

One other finding on a sub-test of the verbal scale is worth reporting, though statistically not significant. On the Digit sub-test a series of numbers have to be repeated first in the order given and then, on another series, in reversed order. Patients nearly always do better in the straight repetition than on the reversal. It had been noticeable three months after the operation that there was an increase in the gap between the number of figures which could be remembered forwards and the number of those remembered backwards. After nine months the gap had widened still further; that is, the difficulty of reversing figures, in contrast with simply remembering them, increased during the year. This is in agreement with the findings of Partridge (1950).

The repetition of digits in reversed order has been shown not to be closely related to general intelligence (G). (Wechsler, 1944.) It appears that failure to repeat digits backwards is often related to difficulties of attention and lack of ability in intellectual work which requires concentrated effort. Thus, again, this may be a reflection of the change in temperament, a change in traits which were reported in detail in the previous chapter.

At three months none of the verbal tests other than Comprehension had shown a marked loss. But after nine months the loss on the Arithmetic sub-test increased, although not quite to the level of significance. The impression given on this test was that the increased loss was due to a greater number of incorrect, impulsive answers: for example, there were failures on the easy questions and passes on the more difficult; thus, again, a change in temperament may be one of the main causes of an apparent loss in ability.

There was one gain on the performance scale which, although it did not reach the level of significance, is worth reporting. Improvement was shown on the Digit Symbol Substitution test. This is a test of the speed and accuracy of the transcription of numbers and symbols, which are associated in a key visible to the patient at all times. The gain on this test was nearer to the level of significance at nine months than at three months. This result suggests an improvement in post-leucotomy patients in carrying out certain routine tasks, even when intelligence is involved.

Porteus Mazes: The Measurement of Non-verbal Intelligence involving Visual Planning

The test of non-verbal intelligence which we selected was Porteus Mazes (Porteus, 1933). This test has been validated by comparing the performance of individuals with assessments obtained on rating scales—as opposed to educational achievement used in the Wechsler scale. Planning and foresight are required to solve these mazes according to Porteus and Kepner (1944) and Porteus and Peters (1947). The test consists of a series of ten mazes which become progressively more difficult. Each maze is printed on a separate sheet and the task is to draw the path that will eventually lead out to the single opening. For each maze successfully completed the patient is credited with points, depending on the number of trials he required to succeed. The sum of the credits received at each year level is transformed into his mental age and the maximum mental age measured by the test is 18 years. The test was administered and scored in the standard way (Porteus, 1933). The last test, labelled the Adult test, was included so as to avoid a 'ceiling' that was too low to show differences in the most intelligent of our patients.

Porteus (1944) and others have shown that when this test is repeated on same individual there is considerable improvement—a gain of as much as two years on the second application of the test has been reported.

A significant loss on this test was found three months after posterior Standard leucotomy; that is, the patients made many more mistakes than they had done prior to the operation. Their behaviour on the mazes may be due to lack of foresight, lack of caution or greater impulsiveness, but it results in a drop in the standard measurements of intelligence on this test—both as regards mental age and the I.Q.

At the second retest nine months after the operation, the loss on the mazes in comparison with pre-operative performance did not quite reach the level of significance.[1] The absence of a significant loss after the longer interval is probably due to the increased practice effect which is known to be pronounced on this particular test; that is, the patients' deficit is somewhat hidden by their having had two previous trials at these same mazes.

There was, however, a significant increase in the number of double mistakes made by the group as a whole both at the three months' and the nine months' investigation. The patients tended to make the same mistake repeatedly after the operation, which did not happen before the operation, suggesting a loss in the ability to learn from errors. If this is one of the effects of leucotomy it may be one reason why in those cases where leucotomy has been performed on children the effects reported have been so poor, the children failing to reach the level of mental development of their contemporaries (Freeman and Watts, 1947; Ritchie Russell, 1948).

Capacity for Generalisation
The Explanation of the Meaning of Proverbs

As a measure of the capacity to generalise we used the six proverbs from the revised Stanford Binet intelligence scale (Terman and Merrill, 1937). The patients' explanations of these proverbs before and after leucotomy were examined independently by the writer, a colleague in the United States and by a psychiatrist. There was considerable agreement between these judges with regard to the individual changes found, and it is clear from their reports that after the operation the patients'

[1] The loss on Porteus Mazes at the second retest is significant in the expected direction. As such a loss has already been found and as it has been noted by other workers (Porteus and Kepner, 1944), it would be permissible to use a one-tail test of significance. This has, however, not been done with any of the other measures and it is undesirable to make an exception on this particular test.

explanations of the proverbs were much more particularised and of that there appeared to be a definite loss in generalisation.

The six proverbs which the patients were asked to interpret before and after the operation will be found in Appendix B. Many examples in the explanations given after the operation indicate a tendency for patients to interpret proverbs too literally. They lack either the capacity or the inclination to generalise to the extent that they did prior to the operation. Sometimes the impression is given that there is a limit to the amount of generalisation they can achieve in respect to any one proverb. They will generalise about one of the items but not about the other. For example, a patient before the operation said 'In order to eat the kernel you must crack the nut' meant 'In order to have the fruits of something you must be prepared to do a little work'; after leucotomy she said, 'You must do a little work to enjoy the kernel.' Before the operation another patient said 'No wind can do him good who steers for no port' meant 'Nothing can help one if one has no aim in life'; after the operation she said, 'If you're not making for anywhere, nothing can do you good.' Before the operation 'We only know the worth of water when the well is dry' meant 'Things are only appreciated when impossible to obtain'; after the operation she said, 'When there is nothing left we know the real worth of things.'

In other cases the amount of generalisation given after the operation is obviously reduced. For example, 'No wind can do him good who steers for no port' was explained before the operation as 'If a man is not attempting to achieve a definite object he does not find anything profitable or of assistance to him'; after the operation the patient wrote, 'If we do not direct our course for some definite destination, no wind or means of transport will benefit us.'

Another said 'Don't judge a book by its cover' meant 'You must delve inside to find out for yourself on things of life rather than go by what you think of outside'; whilst after the operation the explanation given was, 'Don't leave a book by its cover before making a suitable remark thereon. In other words, look (inside the cover to the nature of the contents) before you leap.'

In a few cases generalisation appeared to be completely absent after the operation. For example, before the operation the patient said, 'He who eats the kernel must crack the nut. If you want good things you have got to work for them'; after the operation the patient said, 'If he's going to eat the kernel he'll have to crack the nut first.'

After nine months the interpretation of proverbs showed the same tendency as we have noted after three months. There was no indication that the capacity to generalise had decreased further after the longer period. These findings are of interest in view of Goldstein's (1936) idea that abstract attitudes are primarily affected by leucotomy.

One of the impressions that was gained by both psychologists examining these proverbs was that occasionally the patients achieved a complete answer after the operation but the effort involved appeared to be greater than before the operation. It was as though they arrived by a roundabout route. In these cases we wondered whether perhaps one was witnessing an adaptation to a deficit rather than the deficit itself.

One other noticeable change in the interpretation of proverbs was the patients' tendency to jump from one idea to another far less relevant though in some way associated with the original idea. This may be related to the increased distractibility shown by the patients on other tests.

The total picture obtained suggests that there is a diminished tendency to abstract a general idea from a particular example after the Standard operation of leucotomy, and when attempted is often restricted to only one item in the situation. It appears as though the area of thoughts and ideas previously touched off by one stimulus had shrunk. This diminished tendency to generalise is also shown in the self-description and other essays which are examined later in this chapter. One of the striking changes in these after the operation was the greater particularisation and loss in generalisation, all of which is in agreement with Rylander (1939).

SUMMARY REGARDING INTELLIGENCE TESTS

In contrasting patients on tasks involving intelligence before and three months after leucotomy and again after nine months it has been found that there are losses in verbal tests of intelligence, as opposed to performance tests, in the capacity to generalise, in the ability to learn from errors and in visual planning. There is also a suggestion of greater impulsiveness and a changed attitude towards the social environment. Some of these changes may be partly due to the alterations in temperament described in Chapter II—alterations which might well affect performance on particular intellectual tasks (Petrie, 1949A and B).

Style of Writing
Description of Liked and Disliked People and Self-description

It was decided that the patients' written productions before and after leucotomy should be examined. As changes in social attitudes were of particular interest it was decided to let each patient choose two people to describe, asking only that one of them should be someone liked and the other someone disliked. We also wished to obtain a self-description and hoped that it would be more revealing if the description was in the form 'As others see us'. These essays were done in the patients' own time who wrote as little or as much as they wished. They were told that the papers, as all the other inventories they had filled in, were confidential and that it would be helpful if they could be honest and sincere in their descriptions.

The instructions were as follows:

1. Describe as accurately as you can a person, man or woman, you *like* very much—not his face or appearance, but what he is really like. You may take as long as you wish.

2. Wording as No. 1 except that the person to be described was '*disliked* quite a lot'.

3. Describe yourself as you think you would be seen by the person you describe whom you *like* very much—not your face or appearance, but what you are really like.

4. Wording as No. 3 except that 'the person whom you *dislike* quite a lot' is describing you.

The written productions were examined in order to ascertain whether the loss of generalisation noticed in the proverbs also manifested itself in these essays; whether greater detail and particularisation appeared; whether the more careless use of language (reported later in the chapter) resulted in poorer style; and whether the increased self-esteem shown in self-assessments and estimates of achievement appeared in the essays in the form, for example, of sweeping generalisations; and for any further evidence of changes noted on other tests. In addition to the writer, Dr. Johanna Krout of the Psychological Institute, Chicago, examined all the results independently.

A comparison of essays written before and after showed a clear loss in generalisation and an increase in particularisation. This was shown both with regard to description of personality characteristics and behavioural characteristics.

There was a striking increase in the number of exclamations, rhetorical questions and sweeping general statements; the resulting style appeared bombastic.

After the operation the patients produced more irrelevant statements and appeared more often to run off at a tangent. There was a pronounced increase in the number of references to themselves and particularly noticeable was the manner in which goodness, kindness 'to me' was stressed after leucotomy; the same increased egocentricity was noticed with regard to unkind sentiments.[1]

It had been noticed in the comprehension question on the Wechsler that there was a change in attitude to social standards unconcerned with the immediate environment. In the essays it was noticeable that social qualities were omitted or under-stressed after the operation, except those concerned with behaviour to intimate friends.

The style of writing was poorer and more childish. It was clear that either sentences had been more carelessly put together, or that the same amount of care after the operation produced a result which ran less smoothly and appeared less integrated.

For example, before leucotomy the beginning of the description of a good friend was as follows:

'Perhaps his outstanding characteristic is his personal charm. He is the sort of man who is at home and welcomed in any company, male or female, young or old, and irrespective of the social standing of those with whom he mixes. This is by no means entirely due to an attractive personal appearance or to his winning ways; rather is it due to an innate generosity and

[1] In this connection it is of interest that Harrower Erikson (1940) reported that constriction was shown in the Rorschach records of patients with cerebral tumours. It was suggested that the organism discards all but the most essential types of response with the trauma.

sympathy which will enable him to approach the viewpoint of the other man and so to win the confidence and friendship even of those from whom he differs most strongly.'

After leucotomy the same friend is described as follows:

'He is one of those fortunate people who are almost universally attractive. Of pleasing appearance, he is quite stoutly built and enjoys all the normal forms of sport. He swims well and is good at rugger and tennis. He is a good walker and enjoys the delight of open air life and of taking pleasure in beautiful scenery.'

Other examples of patients' productions will be found in Appendix C.

The essays written by the patients thus afforded us further evidence of the decreased generalisation shown after Standard leucotomy; the accompanying increased particularisation was also manifested. Greater self-esteem was suggested by the more bombastic style; and the lower standards set themselves by patients and perhaps their lowered capacity was shown by the poorer and more childish style of writing. There was also a suggestion of greater egocentricity and of a change in social attitudes.[1]

Perseveration of Ideas

A few of the patients gave answers to questions which indicated some perseveration of ideas. This was found after the operation both at the short and longer period in patients who had not shown any indication of this previously. Thus in answering the vocabulary test where meanings are given for a series of words, a patient used the word 'medicine' in four consecutive descriptions where it did not make sense. Another patient used the word 'qualifications' and did not seem to be able to free himself from it, using it four times in the same sentence. This change is mentioned in passing, as it was not found in the majority of the patients, nor was it frequently manifested in those patients in whom it did appear. It may be an aspect of the same alteration in personality which tended to cause an

[1] Such a wealth of material was provided by the essays that it is hoped to carry out some further investigations on them.

increased number of double mistakes on Porteus mazes; an unwillingness or disinclination to try new approaches to a problem—in this case the problem of expressing oneself.

The Use of Language

One of the interesting findings by the wayside was that the patients displayed a markedly decreased critical attitude towards the use of language after posterior Standard leucotomy. Frequently after leucotomy, but never before, definitions and answers were produced in which common words were misused or new words formed. This was often found on the Wechsler Vocabulary and other verbal tests. In each case the experimenter pretended not to be sure if she had heard correctly; the phrase was then confirmed by the patient. They appeared quite satisfied with their productions and expressed no uneasiness as to their intelligibility. Some of these were borderline cases of language misuse and if found in isolation might be regarded as an original and vivid method of expression. For example, at three months the patients made the following statements:

A woman of average intelligence (verbal I.Q. 109)[1] said 'Hero' is a man who has 'committed skill', 'affliction' is an 'aside' and 'affectation' is people 'pretending what they are not'.

A man with the intelligence level of a superior adult (verbal I.Q. 120) said 'a fable' is 'a far-reaching tale'. On further questioning he stated that he meant 'that it reached far back into history'. He also said that 'dilatory' meant 'doing things in a ship-shop manner' and that 'espionage' meant 'spyism'.

A woman of superior intelligence (verbal I.Q. 121) stated that 'nail' meant 'a metal joiner'; a 'spade' was 'a utensil for gardening'; 'an umbrella is a shade for protection from rain'; 'a sword is an article for killing animals'; 'affliction' meant 'lacking perfection'; 'flout' was 'set against the raising of something'; 'a box' was 'a container usually parallelogram in shape'.

All of which seems to suggest that at any rate three months after leucotomy there is a loss in the finer distinctions of language. It was suggested by some of the psychiatrists to whom this finding was reported that it might be due to the unhealed wounds in the frontal lobes and that it would disappear after the longer period. One was therefore interested to see whether this

[1] Wechsler verbal I.Q. given in each case.

satisfaction with approximate meanings would occur at the second post-leucotomy interview after nine months.

After this further interval definitions and answers were still given which only approximated to the meaning intended by the patients and common words continued to be frequently misused.

For example, a woman of bright intelligence (verbal I.Q. 116) said 'ballast' is 'the weight carried by a ship or other container'; 'a diamond' is 'a carbon compound used in engineering capacites'; 'fur' can be used as 'a wearing apparatus'.

A man of very superior intelligence (verbal I.Q. 143) and with a university degree stated, 'A cat and mouse are alike in that they are both domestic animals.'

A woman of average intelligence (verbal I.Q. 108) said 'a diamond' is 'a worthy jewel'.

There were also more extreme cases of the misuse of language. For example, a woman of average intelligence (verbal I.Q. 103) said 'brave' is 'to show good taste'; 'ballast' is something 'which might enter a balloon or room or anything'.

Another woman of average intelligence (verbal I.Q. 103·5) said, 'Belfry must be your head because they say bats in the belfry.'

Still another stated that 'aseptic' is 'god-like'.

A woman of average intelligence stated that 'Never judge a book by its cover' meant 'Whether the outside be neat or otherwise, it is the internals which will suggest the wealth of the thing.'

There was one case in which an individual of superior intelligence (I.Q. 130) gave the meaning of the word 'belfry' as 'an instrument of defence or attack'. On investigation this proved to be an accurate account of its original etymological meaning.

There were also some examples in the patients' written production of these language phenomena.

A woman of average I.Q. wrote:

'Even medical attentions cannot remove one's inner feelings.'

'An unbearable temper is just another general incident which finally wraps up into your final countenance which to one and all is something to be admired.'

'As long as you regard yourself as equally all right, what does it matter what others think?'

A woman of superior intelligence (with a university degree) wrote:

'She lost her money through old-time lack of sense.'
'She gives large care for her husband's things.'
'She never cared so long as she got attention towards herself.'
'She could not believe that he could be so disregarding to her.'

After nine months she wrote:

'He never referred to his generous actions after arranging them.'
'I shall never forget her straight sitting attitude to sexual illusions.'

A woman of bright intelligence, two years after leucotomy, wrote:

'Belfry is a place where bells are hoisted and kept.'
'Imminent' means 'in danger of happening'.

A woman of superior intelligence, two years after leucotomy, wrote to her doctor:

'Under present decisions possible problems will not arise.'
'I don't care much about me or anyone else, but I know I ought to talk to you if you would tell me possibles for me please.'

The patients' speech appears thus to be slightly out of focus, to be a bit off centre. This is apparent at three months and is, if anything, more frequent at nine months. Moreover, patients after an interval of two years still show the same characteristic. They appear to hit the periphery rather than the bull's eye and show a pronounced inability to find the *mot juste*.

This change in the use of language is reminiscent of some of the speech of schizophrenic patients which has been called by Cameron (1938) 'metonymic distortion'. Such distortion is said to consist of 'the substitution of an approximate but related term or phrase for the more definite term that normal adults would presumably use in the same setting.' Schizophrenic

[1] Further examples of this misuse of language, side by side with the answer to the same question given before the operation, are presented in Appendix C. Some misuse of language was found in all but two of the patients who had been operated on by the Standard method.

language, however, shows much more gross distortion than does the language of these post-leucotomy patients. There are a few examples given by Cameron to make this clear. Thus, his schizophrenic patients stated: 'I am good because brought up right and strictly confidential'; 'I am alive because I was born a human and animal life and normal life'; 'I am alive because you really live physically because you have menus three times a day'; 'Fish can live in the water because it is the natural resource of life'; 'I am good because I think it is best for any physical flesh.'

Other examples do not show so much similarity to the speech of the post-leucotomy patients, but even in the examples quoted the substitution of similar but not equivalent words and phrases is much more evident than in those under examination.

Critchley (1950) has stated that aphasic patients sometimes utter paraphasic errors which distinctly resemble those reported here in leucotomy patients but that the similarity is not close. He suggests that the disorder of language after leucotomy is at a different semantic level than in the case of most aphasias (Critchley, 1948).

There is some similarity between the language of postleucotomy patients and the language of young children. For example, Jonathan, aged 5, talked about a robin which 'noggled with his head', presumably combining 'nod' with 'waggle'. He called rusks 'crusks', combining 'crusts' and 'rusks'. He also talked about 'when you fall awake'.

The child, however, in using such language is not dropping a code of verbal behaviour, for he has not yet fully understood or accepted such a code. The leucotomised patient, prior to the operation, had abided by this code. After the operation he appears to neglect the standards he had previously set himself with regard to exactitude in verbal expression.

There are at least two possible theories to account for this change in the use of language after posterior Standard leucotomy. One is that the patient is incapable of selecting and recognising the right word or phrase. The other is that he is displaying a carelessness and lack of conscientiousness in the selection of words. There is no evidence to prove definitely which of these two theories is correct; both processes may be at work. But there is evidence in the performance of patients on a variety of tests that they are more careless after leucotomy. We have pointed out in the previous chapter that they tend after the operation to make more mistakes in both manual and mental tasks, and also tackle these tasks at a much greater speed than they did before the operation. It is reasonable to suggest that the increased tendency to make mistakes, the lowered standards of accuracy and achievement, are evident in their use of language; in fact, that this finding is but one aspect of the more general one that patients after leucotomy tend to be less accurate, tend to be more hurried, set themselves lower standards and are more satisfied with a poorer performance. But this does not exclude the possibility that posterior Standard leucotomy may occasion an incapacity to recognise the exact area of meaning of a word.

It was thought that some light might be thrown on the interpretation of this change in use of language by presenting to a patient—who had been operated—the pre-leucotomy reply to certain questions, side by side with the post-leucotomy reply showing the misuse of language. We prepared such a set of examples and decided to show them to a highly intelligent postleucotomy patient—M. A., with a first-class university degree—for her to assess the correctness of the various answers. We attempted to obtain both a judgment as to which of the answers was correct and an explanation of what was wrong with the incorrect answers.

The impression given by this patient was that she did not discriminate clearly between the answers in which language was correctly used and those in which it was incorrectly used. Moreover, when she did criticise an answer it was for a relatively irrelevant reason. For example, the question 'How are a cat and a mouse alike?' was answered by one patient before the operation, 'They keep up at night looking for food; both on alert at night; quick.' After the operation the patient said, 'They are seekers, usually for their food.' M. A., confronted with these two answers, approved the second answer and queried the first. She criticised the first description suggesting that cats are not always alert at night, 'at least not perpetually since many cats sleep through much of the night.' She agreed that both were quick in their movements.

A diamond had been described as 'a jewel' before the operation and as 'a worthy jewel' afterwards. M. A. looked at these two answers and said hesitantly, 'I don't like the word "worthy" very much there.' She did not, however, suggest that it was using 'worthy' improperly, that it had another meaning or that 'valuable' might have been a more suitable word or a phrase with 'worth' in it. Another patient had said after the operation that it was right to choose candidates for Civil Service examinations because 'it makes people unpolitical'. The comment of M. A. on this was, 'It doesn't make people unpolitical; it gets people with best examinee brain.'

A post-leucotomy patient had said that a 'letter' was 'something you send to friends which is really a collection of words.' Confronted with this M. A. said, 'Something omitted here; it should be collection of words sending meaning.' Another patient had said after leucotomy that 'letter' was an 'independent unit of the alphabet'. M. A. said about this, 'She is being awfully clever; it would be better if she said one member of the alphabet.'

One patient had said after leucotomy that 'bad' meant 'not too good'. M. A. suggested that this was 'not sufficiently accurate'.

'Nuisance' had been described by a post-leucotomy patient as being 'a bit of a bother and a humbug—one as well as the other.' This had been approved as correct and satisfactory by M. A.

One patient said that nitroglycerine was 'used for inventing—I think an explosive—you've got to find out these things.' M. A. studied this post-leucotomy production and said, 'It was discovered some time ago, I believe; she needn't say "used for inventing".'

There were other examples which suggested that for this post-leucotomy patient the division between the correct and incorrect use of language was not clear, even when she was confronted with both types of answer to the same question. It is of interest that she was looking for mistakes; she had been told to mark with a cross those answers that would not pass. In spite of this some were overlooked; others were vaguely commented on, but not in a manner that showed a clear idea in the patient's mind of the meaning of the misused word.

Though further research would be needed to confirm this, the criticisms and explanations given by this patient suggest that it is not purely carelessness that has determined the misuse of language shown after posterior Standard leucotomy by patients. There is some indication that the 'aura' of words has changed for them. This, of course, is different from person to person, but here it has become different in the same person. It is possible that other defects shown by these patients are related to this change in the precise meaning of words. This language phenomenon is of particular interest in view of the confirmation of the existence of Broca's expressive speech centre in Area 44 (Penfield and Rasmussen, 1950).

The writer has found that in examining patients who have not undergone leucotomy but have had some type of brain injury which has involved the frontal lobes, comparable changes in the use of language do occasionally appear. For example, there was a patient of high intelligence who had been injured during the war and as a result had the frontal-parietal area repaired with a tantalum plate, and was known to have extensive damage of his left frontal lobe (reported by Osmond, 1950). This man gave practically no indication of organic deterioration on all the classical measures. He did, however, state that 'a belfry was *a garage in which the bells were kept.*' This would have been in keeping if it had been said by a post-leucotomy patient.

Another head injury patient, of superior intelligence and with a university education, did show many classical signs of deterioration. In addition he stated that 'an umbrella consisted of a handle which contained a spindle and ribs which contained a silk cover'; and 'bad' was a word which meant 'evil and had a deleterious effect on those who used it.'

There is thus the possibility that this language phenomenon may be characteristic of patients who have had some injury to the part of the frontal lobe involved in a posterior Standard operation.[1] If further results show this to be the case it would be useful to develop a list of questions which tend to elicit answers demonstrating this phenomenon. For instance, it will be

[1] Since writing the above a report has appeared in the *Lancet* of the effect of a bullet wound through both frontal lobes (Slorach, 1951). The writer mentions in passing the patient's difficulty in finding nouns and quotes his description of the nurses as 'sugar-iced people'. This is in keeping with the peculiar speech forms I have reported after Standard posterior leucotomy.

noticed that in the examples reported the definitions of 'belfry' and 'ballast' appear frequently to produce approximate rather than exact use of words, and it may be found that there is a relationship between the stage of life when the word was learnt and its tendency to be misused after the operation.

After posterior Standard leucotomy we have found many examples of the approximate use of language, which persists years after the operation and is to be found both in writing and speaking. There is some evidence that this failing may be found specifically in injury of the more posterior parts of the frontal lobes. It may be caused partly by the change in temperament involving greater carelessness and lower standards found in patients after posterior leucotomy. There is also evidence that there may be contributory factors in the patient's inability to recognise the right word, apart from his unwillingness to be bothered to find it.

CHAPTER FOUR

THE EFFECT OF BILATERAL AND UNILATERAL ANTERIOR ROSTRAL LEUCOTOMY ON PERSONALITY

IN the last two chapters we described the changes in personality found after the posterior Standard operation on the frontal lobes. These effects were examined three months after and again nine months after the operation. It was found that these changes occurred in the sphere of temperament, character and intelligence and that the pattern of orectic personality changes—that is, in temperament and character—was in line with our main hypothesis of a decrease in neuroticism and a decrease in introversion.

If these results were indicative of interference with the functions of intact frontal lobes as a whole, one would expect that a more anterior operation would result in changes which were of a similar pattern to those found in the posterior Standard operation. If, however, the function of different parts of the frontal lobe was clearly defined, it would be expected that a change in the operation, a change in the position of the incision, would result in considerable difference to the type of personality change found. I had an opportunity of examining a series of patients who had the open Rostral operation—the more anterior incision—used by Mr. McKissock.[1] The cases were bilaterally operated as in the Standard procedure. The personality changes are reported in this chapter. In addition to the changes after the bilateral anterior operation, the effects of unilateral leucotomy on the left and right frontal lobes will be described.

The opportunity to examine patients with a more anterior incision resulted from therapeutic considerations. After the Standard operation, in some of the patients, the personality had changed

[1] Details of operative techniques were given in Chapter I.

too much. It was also hoped that a more anterior operation might avoid some of the less desirable effects, whilst it succeeded in its therapeutic purpose of relieving the neurotic illness.

It had also been noted that there was considerable variation in the effectiveness of the closed operation. It was thought that possibly the open operation would avoid that difference in effectiveness dependent on the variation in the fibres cut in the closed procedure. This variation is partly due to individual difference in the architecture of the brain, as in the closed leucotomy the neurosurgeon, although making his incision at the same point of the skull, has no check as to what precisely is underneath the bone. In an open operation the neurosurgeon can be somewhat more certain as to the exact position of his incision (Le Beau, 1942).

It was hoped by means of objective tests to contribute to the understanding of the effect of this anterior operation. If the tests are sufficiently sensitive we would expect, moreover, that in comparing the posterior Standard with the anterior Rostral operation, differences would be apparent on at least some of our measurements. Greater variation in test changes after the closed than after the open operation would also be expected.

In the investigation of Standard patients it had been found that most of the changes were present at three months, but were more accentuated after the longer interval, and that some changes only showed themselves clearly after the longer period. It was decided to examine Rostral patients before and approximately six months after the operation. The investigations were identical with those carried out on Standard patients. A few additional tests were used, however, in an attempt to gain more understanding of some of the findings on Standard patients. As most of the tests have already been described (see also Appendix A), only the briefest reference to them will be made in this chapter. The number of the test in the Appendix will, however, be indicated, so that no difficulty should be experienced by the reader in referring to the description of administration and scoring.

The type of patient selected for this operation was, as far as possible, the same as that for the Standard operation. During a certain period every patient on whom it was decided to carry out a leucotomy was given the Rostral operation instead of the Standard. There was no indication that the two groups of patients differed in any significant way prior to the operation. They had the same type of treatment prior to the operation and their stay in hospital was of comparable length.

Fifteen patients who had undergone bilateral Rostral were examined. Two of these were males and thirteen were females. Thirteen of the patients were married, but two of these were separated; two patients were unmarried.

Five (33%) were diagnosed as depressives;

Three (20%) were diagnosed as anxiety cases;

Three (20%) were diagnosed as obsessionals;

One (7%) was diagnosed as a hysteric;

Three (20%) were of mixed diagnosis, which included one case of anorexia nervosa.

Of the two males one was a case of anxiety and one was obsessional.

The average age of the bilateral patients was 43·21 years (range 27 to 58). The average Wechsler I.Q. was 100·43 (range 71 to 125).

Two patients had been to a university; six had attended secondary schools and two of these had further technical training. The technical education of two patients had followed attendance at elementary schools. The remaining five had attended elementary schools only.

After the operation one patient returned to work as a buyer in a large firm, and others as a bookkeeper, chef, Civil Service clerk and a tailor's assistant. Two worked as shorthand-typists. There were also several housewives who resumed their duties at home; before their marriage some of these had been shop assistants, factory workers and domestic employees.

Methods of analysis used

We have compared scores on tests before and after the operation and have noted those differences which are significant at the 5% level of probability; that is, we are reporting as significant those changes which would occur less than once in twenty by chance.[1] Statistical details will be found in Appendix B.

[1] In the case of the Rostral operation the hypothesis was based on the findings in two repeat tests after the Standard operation. It was therefore considered correct to use a one-tail test of significance in working out our probability level.

CHANGES AFTER BILATERAL ROSTRAL LEUCOTOMY ON TESTS RELATED TO NEUROTICISM

1. *Suggestibility*

The Rostral patients showed a change in Body Sway suggestibility. There was a marked decrease in suggestibility, the patients swaying much less after the operation than they had before.

2. *Disposition Rigidity*
Perseveration Test

There was a change after the operation in the patients' behaviour on a task involving alternating activity. They found it easier to shift from one type of activity to another, from writing the figures 2, 3, 4 in the usual manner and then with reversed strokes; that is, they had lower perseveration scores.

3. *Manual Dexterity*

The highest score achieved in a series of trials on the Track Tracer was significantly higher after the operation than before.

4. *Speed of Writing*

The speed of writing words (ready) and figures (2, 3, 4) had increased after the operation.

5. *Self-criticism*

There was a decrease in the number of undesirable character traits ascribed to themselves by patients after the operation.

6. *Smoothness of Work Curves*

No significant changes were found in the smoothness of work curves.[1]

SUMMARY: NEUROTICISM

It will thus be seen that of the five variables related to neuroticism, the Rostral patients showed significant changes in the direction of a decrease in neuroticism. These changes were all present after the Standard operation.

[1] It should be pointed out that through some technical difficulty we were not able to obtain complete records of one of these smoother work curves, viz. the speed of tapping in 4 quarter-minutes.

CHANGES AFTER BILATERAL ROSTRAL LEUCOTOMY ON TESTS
RELATED TO INTROVERSION

7. *Speed and Accuracy*

a. Accuracy

On a few of the tests there was an increase in the number of mistakes made. This was the case on Porteus Mazes, although the increase was just below the level of significance. No loss in mental age and I.Q. was found on this test.[1] It is interesting that in spite of this, if the number of mistakes is calculated irrespective of whether they occur on the easier or more difficult mazes, we were able to show the tendency of patients after operation to be more inaccurate on this as on other tasks. (In estimating mental age and I.Q., mistakes in easier tasks are the most highly penalised.)

An increased number of mistakes was made on the Track Tracer both on the individual trials and in the total on all trials. This, however, did not reach the level of significance. The ratio of speed to mistakes on the individual trials had also decreased, but fell short of significance. There was, in addition, an increase in the number of errors in the test of concentration.

b. Speed

The patients completed the course on the Track Tracer more quickly than before the operation. This was shown on the trials considered individually and on the total of all trials. They were quicker after the operation than before in completing Porteus Mazes. The speed of decision had increased, in that the patients took less time to decide how they would rate a series of jokes. The total time taken by the patient on the Wechsler Arithmetic test had decreased.

What is important in these four results is that on totally different tasks—involving respectively manual dexterity, diligent planning in a non-verbal test of intelligence, decisions on attitudes to a series of jokes and the solution of problems in mental arithmetic—the patients were taking much less time after the operation than they had before.

From which it may be seen that the results provide an indication that the patient is tending to make more mistakes after the

[1] Results of Porteus Mazes are reported in detail under Intellectual Aspects.

operation but this change is not so obvious as is the increase in speed.

8. *Tendency towards Self-blame: Intropunitive Reactions to Incapacities*

The self-blame inventory was used which had demonstrated changes after Standard leucotomy. An estimate of his unpleasant characteristics was provided by the patient; he was then asked whether he blamed himself for these characteristics and if so whether 'exceedingly', 'very much' or 'a little'.

The patient's attitude had changed after the operation. He blamed himself for fewer characteristics and for such as he did the intensity of his self-blame had decreased.

9. *Attitude to Time*

The answers given by the patients to eight questions about their attitude to the past, present and future indicated that after the anterior operation they were less oriented to the past and more to the present and future. Thus 36% more of the patients thought most about the present after the operation, 19% ceased to find in the past their main source of happiness and 38% more of the patients became most interested in the future.

10. *Humour*
a. *Appreciation of Sex Humour*

The rating of the twenty-five jokes by the Rostral patients reproduced some of the tendencies found in the Standard posterior groups, but to a slighter extent. Two of the sex jokes which were found to go up in rating, both three months after the posterior operation and again at nine months, were also found to be going up in rating after the anterior operation. Of the remaining sex jokes which did not show an all-over increase in rating, a few nevertheless jumped to the category 'extremely amusing' for some of the Rostral patients. The neutral jokes which moved down at both Standard retests showed a tendency in the same direction after the anterior operation. One of these neutral jokes was the only one to come down three categories in comparison with the pre-operative rating; and two of the jokes, having been 'amusing' before the operation, became 'not amusing' afterwards. (This has to be evaluated against the general tendency for fewer jokes to be considered 'not amusing' after the operation.) There is thus a tendency for sex jokes, in comparison with neutral jokes, to go up in rating.

b. Change in Attitude to Pictorial Humour

The change in the rating of twenty-five jokes was a decrease (almost significant) in the number of jokes found 'not amusing'. There was also a suggestive increase in the number of jokes found in the category 'slightly amusing'.

Ratio of Verbal Intelligence to Performance Intelligence Scores

After Rostral leucotomy the patients had a higher performance score in relation to their verbal score, on the Wechsler scale, than prior to the operation.

11. *Endurance*

We gave two tests of endurance. One was the leg test which we had used with Standard patients; the other was the grip on a dynamometer which has been shown to be closely correlated with other measures of endurance (Himmelweit and Petrie, 1951). On the dynamometer the patient had slightly lower scores, although not significantly, after the operation than before. On the leg test, however, there was no decrease in endurance as had been the case after the Standard operation.

12. *Level of Aspiration*

The various measures which we used do not show after this type of anterior Rostral operation a lowering of goals suggested after the Standard operation. With regard to judgments of time the patients overrated their performance; this change did not quite reach the level of significance though it is in harmony with decreased introversion (Himmelweit, 1947). That is, the patients tended to think that they had completed the series of trials on the Track Tracer more quickly than in fact they had.

SUMMARY: INTROVERSION

The pattern of changes on the majority of these variables is the same as that found after the Standard operation, and indicates a decrease in introversion (Petrie, 1949c). Only the direction and the significance of the change has been reported here. Differences in the extent of the changes after these two operations will be discussed in Chapter V.

CHANGES AFTER BILATERAL ROSTRAL LEUCOTOMY ON MISCELLANEOUS PERSONALITY TESTS

13. *Fluctuation or Reversal of Perspective*

After the Rostral operation the rate of willed fluctuation of an ambiguous figure (the Necker Cube) had increased, whilst the rate of unwilled fluctuation had not changed. The difference between the rate of willed and unwilled fluctuation had also increased.

14. *Concentration and Distractibility*

The patients improved slightly in concentration after the operation on a test involving figures. The difference between concentration with and without the distraction did not suggest an increase in distractibility after the anterior operation as had been shown after the Standard operation. There was, however, a significant increase in the relapses on the test of distractibility; that is, the output was more uneven in this test than it had been prior to the operation. This suggests that in some ways the distraction may be more potent after the operation than before.

15. *Time Judgment*

The patients changed in their judgment of a period of a minute. Their estimation was longer after the operation than before. The same suggestive tendency appeared in the judgment of a period of 15 seconds.

16. *Fluency*

No significant changes were found on the two tests of fluency, although on both somewhat greater fluency was shown after the operation.

17. *Persistence at a Task*

The patient was given an opportunity to spend as long as he liked and be as productive as he wished at a task of word building. After the anterior Rostral operation he tended to stay longer at this task and to be more productive, although the change was not significant.

18. *Attitude to Illness*

The patients were asked before and after the operation

whether they considered themselves to be ill, and if so whether they though they would get better. There was considerable qualification in the answers to these two questions after the Rostral operation and our analysis was therefore carried out to include groups who believed that they were still a little ill and those who were hopeful—though not certain—about getting better. There was a clear tendency after the anterior operation for patients to believe themselves to be better, though this was less obvious than after the posterior operation. Nine considered they had improved as a result of the operation. Of six patients who considered themselves to be ill, three were no longer hesitant or doubtful about the improvement in their health which was going to take place in the future. It would seem that the subjective belief of a patient is either that his health has greatly improved as a result of the Rostral operation or that it will improve if given time.

SUMMARY: MISCELLANEOUS TESTS

The constellation of changes after the anterior bilateral Rostral operation on miscellaneous personality tests is the same as that found after the posterior Standard operation.

ADDITIONAL PERSONALITY TESTS WHICH HAVE ONLY BEEN USED ON ROSTRAL PATIENTS

A few additional tests were used on Rostral patients in order to contribute to our understanding of the personality changes.

19. *Worries*

An inventory was used which consisted of a list of items about which people might worry. The patient was asked to underline 'anything which he worried about at this period of his life'. There was a suggestive decrease in the number of worries after the operation, but not reaching the level of significance.

20. *Interests*

An inventory consisting of items in which people might be interested was presented to each patient and he was asked to underline 'everything in which he was interested at this time of his life'. The patient after the operation found more things interesting than before the operation, but this was only a slight increase and is reported primarily because it contrasts with the suggestive decrease in the number of worries. It has been shown that individuals who are successful in certain professions under-line more items in this interest questionnaire than do those who are unsuccessful (Petrie and Powell, 1950 and 1951).

21. *Annoyances*

In a list of annoyances which the patient marked before and after the operation it was found that there were no suggestive differences.[1]

22. *Cattell's Self-inventory*

The results of numerous investigations using self-inventories —on a large variety of subjects—were analysed by Cattell. He extracted two factors, C (neurotic general emotionality) and F (surgency), which are remarkably similar to Eysenck's factors of neuroticism and introversion.

Cattell (1946) has shown that the factors of neuroticism (C) and of introversion (F) are each associated with five charac-teristics in a self-inventory. The *neurotic* regards himself as:

1. Frequently in low spirits.
2. Lonesome even with friends.
3. Frequently grouchy.
4. Getting easily discouraged.
5. Unadjusted to life.

Questions regarding these five traits were answered by eleven bilateral Rostral patients before and after their operation. Some change was shown on each question, and all changes were in the direction of a decrease in neuroticism; that is, these traits were less frequently ascribed to themselves by patients after Rostral leucotomy. The most pronounced change was the increase in the number of patients who denied that they were frequently in low spirits.

The *introvert* in a self-inventory regards himself as:

1. Often just miserable for no reason.
2. Prone to worry over possible misfortunes.

[1] The Worries, Interests and Annoyances inventories were adaptations of the Pressey X/O test.

3. Having frequent ups and downs in mood.
4. Meditative and introspective.
5. Unable to relax; not carefree.

Changes were found in eleven patients on each of these, with the exception of Item 4. All changes were in the direction of a decrease in introversion; that is, these characteristics were less frequently ascribed to themselves by patients after Rostral leucotomy.

The change on questions related to introversion was slightly more obvious than on those related to neuroticism. It has been reported that Rostral patients change less than Standard patients on other tests related to introversion; the clear alteration in this direction in the self-inventory is therefore of great interest.

THE EFFECT OF BILATERAL ROSTRAL LEUCOTOMY ON INTELLECTUAL ASPECTS OF PERSONALITY

Wechsler Bellevue Scale of Intelligence: Verbal and Performance Tests

No loss was found after the operation in the Wechsler (Form II) verbal I.Q., performance I.Q. or the total I.Q. based on four performance and four verbal tests. Indeed, on the Arithmetic and Similarities sub-test there is a significant improvement. All these results contrast strikingly with those found after Standard leucotomy.

Two findings on the sub-tests, however, were reminiscent of the behaviour of Standard patients. One was the improvement on the Digit Symbol test; the other the suggestive increased difference between the memory for digits forward and backward, patients finding it relatively more difficult to reverse digits.

Comprehension sub-test

There was no significant change on the Comprehension sub-test as a whole. A loss had been present after the posterior Standard operation.

The scores on answers to the ten questions making up this sub-test were analysed. On two of them there were significant changes after the operation. These were an improvement in answering 'Why is cotton used in making cloth?' and a loss in answering 'Why should a promise be kept?' It will be noticed that the contrast between these two questions suggests that the patients are showing a loss in social attitudes and a gain in supplying factual information. The change after the Standard operation had suggested that the five questions showing a loss group themselves to cover an area concerned with social attitudes to the non-immediate environment. It is of interest that, in spite of the fact that anterior Rostral patients did not have lower I.Q.s, nor lower scores on the Comprehension sub-test, as did the posterior Standard patients, we can still find a trace of the differential response to questions involving social attitudes and factual knowledge after the operation. The change, of course, is more muted and on this particular test is shown by statistically significant differences—in a contrasted direction—on two questions.

Porteus Mazes

No change was found in the Standard scoring of performance on Porteus Mazes; that is, the patient's mental age and I.Q. on this test did not drop significantly. We did, however, note a suggestive increase in the number of double mistakes made in completing the mazes. We have already reported that the speed with which they were completed was much greater than before the operation.

Capacity for Generalisation
The Explanation of the Meaning of Proverbs

The patients were given six proverbs of the Stanford Binet scale to explain. The interpretations did not indicate a lack of generalisation or poorer performance after the operation. Sometimes it was found that the explanation of the proverb was more satisfactory before Rostral leucotomy; in others it was more clearly expressed afterwards.

The Use of Language

At least six hours were spent in examining each patient after the operation and in addition they produced a considerable quantity of written material. There was no indication, however, of a change in the use of language; words were not misused, approximate meanings were not given in definitions and words

74

were not stretched to cover an area for which they were not currently intended. Thus, after the anterior Rostral operation there was no indication of the less critical use of language or of greater carelessness in the choice of words, as was shown after the posterior Standard operation.

What is important in all this is that on two comprehensive tests of intelligence, as well as in the interpretation of proverbs and in the use of language, we found no loss after the Rostral operation as had been present after the Standard operation.

The more anterior operation shows the same pattern of changes as the posterior operation in the orectic aspects of personality—in the sphere of temperament and character. There is a decrease on five traits related to neuroticism and a decrease on five traits related to introversion. The two operations differ fundamentally, however, in their effect on intellectual aspects of personality. The losses present after posterior Standard leucotomy are absent after anterior Rostral leucotomy (Petrie, 1949C, 1950A&B). The interpretation of these similarities and differences will be postponed until we have considered in Chapter V the difference in the extent of the changes following on the two operations.

A COMPARISON OF RIGHT AND LEFT ROSTRAL OPERATIONS (ANTERIOR INCISION)

It is, of course, possible that the localisation of functions in the frontal lobes might be related to the position of the incision considered from the left as opposed to the right side. It was therefore desirable in addition to examining personality changes after bilateral anterior operations, to note what changes occurred in patients on whom only the left or only the right sides had been operated, referred to in the text as the left and right group respectively.

Four patients with left Rostral operations were compared with four patients with right Rostral operations. These were all right-handed females. Five of the patients were married.

Those operated on the right frontal lobe were diagnosed as three cases of depression and one of anxiety. Of those operated on the left three were of mixed diagnosis and one was an obsessional. They were seen approximately two months after the operation.[1]

The tests and procedure were identical with that described above for the bilateral Rostral. These numbers are so small that only the general trend will be reported and the effect of left and right operations will be compared with that of the bilateral anterior Rostral operation.[2]

THE EFFECT OF LEFT AND RIGHT OPERATIONS ON MEASUREMENTS RELATED TO NEUROTICISM

1. *Suggestibility*

The pattern of changes on the three scores on this test were similar after the left operation to that found after the bilateral operation; the right, although dissimilar, did show a clear decrease in suggestibility.

2. *Disposition Rigidity*

On tests of perseveration neither the left nor right Rostrals corresponded to the pattern of changes after the bilateral operation, although both groups showed a decrease in Disposition Rigidity on one of the tests.

3. *Highest Score on the Track Tracer*

There was an improvement in the highest score attained on the Track Tracer in a series of trials after both operations. The left operation showed greater consistency in its effect on this variable than did the right.

4. *Speed of Writing*

The increased speed of writing was shown by the left patients

[1] The procedure in the anterior Rostral originally was that the operation on one side of the brain was carried out first and then after an interval of approximately two months the operation on the other side. The neurosurgeon alternated in the side where he made his first incision. The improvement in four of these patients was so great that a second operation was not carried out. Two of these had been operated on the left, two on the right. At a later stage it was arranged that the operation on the two sides should be carried out under the one anaesthetic, in order to save time and hospital beds, and we then were not able to continue to examine the effect of the unilateral operation.

[2] Statistical tables of changes after left and right operations have not been included because of the paucity of numbers.

and not by the right. This was noticeable both in writing figures and words.

5. *Self-criticism*

The decrease in self-criticism shown by the left group was more pronounced than that shown by the right.

6. *Smothness of Work Curves*

This was omitted as no change was found after the bilateral incision.

CHANGES AFTER LEFT AND RIGHT OPERATIONS ON MEASURE-MENTS RELATED TO INTROVERSION

7. *Speed and Accuracy*

a. *Accuracy*

On the series of Porteus Mazes more mistakes were made after operations on the left side but not after operations on the right side.

There was no agreement between left and right pattern and bilateral pattern with regard to mistakes on the Track Tracer considered individually and in all trials. A comparison, however, of the ratio of speed to mistakes indicated that the left were nearer to the bilateral pattern than were the right. In a test of concentration more mistakes were made by the left group whilst the right group did not increase their score.

b. *Speed*

Less time was taken to complete the set of Porteus Mazes after both types of operation. The decrease, however, was more consistent after the left than after the right operation.

The speed of decision had increased after both types of operation. Those operated on the left, however, showed a more consistent and pronounced increase than those operated on the right.

Less time was taken over the Wechsler Mental Arithmetic test after both operations. Those operated on the left showed a more consistent decrease than those operated on the right.

The time taken on the Track Tracer trials—both considered individually and over the series of trials—had decreased after the operation on the left side. No change on individual trials was shown in the operation on the right side.

8. *The Tendency towards Self-blame*

The total number of items in the self-blame inventory for

which patients blamed themselves after the operation had decreased consistently and obviously in the left but not the right Rostrals. The decrease in intensity of self-blame was also slightly more consistent and pronounced in the left than in the right.

9. *Attitude to Time*

The pattern of change in the group operated on the left in their attitude to the past, present and future more closely resembled that of the bilateral group than did the right. Moreover, four of the differences in the bilateral group had reached the level of significance; these were found in the left group but not in the right.

10. *Attitude to Sex Humour*

No clear change was apparent in either the right or left patients following operation.

CHANGES AFTER LEFT AND RIGHT OPERATIONS ON MISCELLANEOUS PERSONALITY TESTS

In the following measurements the pattern of personality changes on the left was closer than the right to that of the bilaterals:

An increase in fluency was shown after the left operation on the two fluency tests—but not after the right.

Increased productivity in a test of persistence at a task was more consistent and definite in the left than in the right.

The total output in the test of concentration had increased in the left and not in the right.

The left showed more pronounced variations in output than the right in a test of distractibility.

Increased fluctuation with effort as compared with fluctuation without effort was shown by the left and not the right.

A survey of the detailed test results suggests strongly that, on measures related to orectic aspects of personality, there is a tendency for an incision on the left side to have an effect closer to a bilateral operation than one on the right side. This is particularly clearly shown in the measurements related to neuroticism and those related to introversion on which our original hypothesis was based; that is, left Rostrals show a more pronounced decrease in tests related to neuroticism and a more pronounced decrease in tests related to introversion than do right Rostrals.

CHANGES AFTER LEFT AND RIGHT OPERATIONS ON INTELLECTUAL ASPECTS OF PERSONALITY

The Wechsler Bellevue Scale of Intelligence: Verbal and Performance Tests

The direction of the change in left Rostrals on the verbal I.Q., performance I.Q. and full-scale Wechsler I.Q. is the same as that of bilateral Rostrals. This similarity in the pattern of changes is not present in right Rostrals.

Comprehension sub-test: analysis of answers given to ten questions

Two significant differences were found after the bilateral Rostral operation in answers given to the Comprehension questions. One of these was a loss; one was a gain. Left Rostrals show the same tendency on the same two questions more clearly than do the right Rostrals.

Porteus Mazes

There is no noticeable contrast between the behaviour of left and right Rostrals on Porteus Mazes. Both show a slight loss in mental age and I.Q.

SUMMARY: LEFT AND RIGHT OPERATIONS

On intellectual measures as well as on personality measures there is a strong tendency for left Rostrals to have a pattern of change closely allied to that of bilateral Rostrals; this similarity of pattern is less pronounced in right Rostrals. Changes in personality, therefore, suggest that the incision on the left may be contributing more than the incision on the right to the effect of bilateral leucotomy. This poses the question of the function of left as opposed to the right intact frontal lobe.

The change in personality after the bilateral anterior operation will be contrasted with those after the bilateral posterior operation in the next chapter.

CHAPTER FIVE

A COMPARISON OF THE EFFECTS OF ANTERIOR ROSTRAL AND POSTERIOR STANDARD LEUCOTOMY

SIGNIFICANCE OF DIFFERENCE BETWEEN STANDARD AND ROSTRAL PATIENTS

An analysis was carried out of the difference between the effects on personality of the Standard and Rostral operations to ascertain on which measurements the differences reached the level of significance, and whether there was any support for the hypothesis that the Rostral operation caused less marked changes in personality than the Standard. The 't' test was used to measure the significance of the difference between the two sets of scores (see footnote, Chapter I, page 14).

It will be remembered that the investigations after the posterior Standard operation were carried out three months after and nine months after the operation. In the case of the Rostral anterior operation the investigations were carried out but once, six months after the operation. Changes after the Rostral were compared with those after both the early and the later Standard investigation.

As might be expected from the report of the changes in the posterior and anterior operations the significant differences were primarily found on tests of intelligence. Some of the differences between the two operations on intellectual measures not only reached the level of significance but were above the 1% level of probability. This was true of verbal I.Q. (Wechsler scale) in the comparison of the Rostral with the Standard both at three months and nine months after the operation ($t=4 \cdot 02$ at three months and $3 \cdot 01$ at nine months), and of the full-scale I.Q. at three months ($t=3 \cdot 01$). (Although still above the level of

80

significance, the difference in the full-scale I.Q.—that is, eight verbal and performance tests—had dropped at the nine months' retest ($t=2 \cdot 36$).) The third score giving a striking difference between the two types of operation was the Comprehension sub-test ($t=3 \cdot 09$ at three months and $2 \cdot 19$ at nine months).

There was also a significant difference between the two operations in their effect on the scores of the Arithmetic ($t=2 \cdot 66$ and $2 \cdot 78$) and Similarities sub-test of the Wechsler scale ($t=3 \cdot 02$ and $2 \cdot 94$). All these scores, it will be remembered, are in the direction of a greater loss in the Standard posterior operation than in the Rostral anterior operation.

A significant difference was found to exist between the two operations on answers to two of the ten questions on the Comprehension sub-test. These were what the patient should do if he saw a train approaching a broken track ($t=2 \cdot 70$ and $2 \cdot 39$), and also why he thought it was generally better to give money to an organised charity than to a street beggar ($t=2 \cdot 06$ and $2 \cdot 27$). The Rostral group answered the questions more satisfactorily. These were two of the questions involving social attitudes on which a significant loss was found after the Standard operation. Although there is evidence to suggest that a change in social attitude is also present to a slight extent after the Rostral operation, it is clear that the change after the anterior operation does not appear to affect the area covered by the two questions mentioned here.

In comparing the Rostral operation with the Standard at the three months' follow-up, a significant difference was found with regard to mental age and I.Q. on Porteus Mazes ($t=2 \cdot 14$). Standard patients showed a significant loss; Rostral patients did not. The difference, however, disappeared when the Rostrals were compared with the nine months' follow-up of the Standard patients ($t=0 \cdot 93$).

It will be remembered that the loss on the mazes at the later Standard follow-up was not significant. This result, therefore, may be partly due—in the case of the Standard patients—to the effect of extra practice acquired by a third testing with the mazes.

There were no significant differences between the two operations in their effect on measurements related to neuroticism.

On traits related to introversion-extroversion there were two significant differences between the operations. The loss in endurance on the leg test was not present in the Rostral patients but had been found in Standard patients. The difference between the two operations on this test reached the level of significance ($t=2.76$ and 2.47)[1]

One of the five scores on the test of self-blame (blaming 'a little') was used more by the Rostrals than the Standards (at the second retest only) and the difference reached the level of significance ($t=0.10$ and 2.25). But this may not be due to a difference between the two types of incision but to the following cause: there was a very marked decrease between the Standard follow-up at three months and nine months with regard to the number of items for which patients blamed themselves 'a little'. As the Rostral follow-up was carried out at six months it may be that the full change on this measure—shown only at nine months in the Standards—had not yet manifested itself. This seems probable, as it is one of the very few scores on which a pronounced change is shown between three months and nine months on Standard patients.

In comparing the effect of these two operations on orectic personality tests it was found that on measures related to neuroticism there are no significant differences, on measures related to diminished introversion there is one (leg persistence). With regard to intellectual measures, however, there is a marked difference in the effect of the two operations. This was particularly noticeable on the verbal I.Q. and the Comprehension, Similarities and Arithmetic sub-tests of the Wechsler scale. An analysis of the ten questions on the Comprehension sub-test indicated that although a change in social attitude was present in Rostral patients, it was not as striking as that found in Standard patients.

[1] This particular test is known to be related to both neuroticism and extroversion but more strongly to the latter (Petrie, 1948A; Himmelweit and Petrie, 1951). If a patient becomes less neurotic, one would expect the scores to go up to a certain extent; if the patient becomes less introverted, one would expect the scores to go down. Later in the chapter it will be reported that the Rostral operation causes a less marked change than the Standard on tests related to introversion; it may be that on this particular test the decrease in endurance is hidden by the effect of a change in neuroticism.

EFFECTS OF DIFFERENT OPERATIONS

Although the pattern of changes in tests of temperament and character was the same after the Rostral and Standard operations, there was a difference in the extent of these changes.

Changes (mean difference) on tests related to diminished neuroticism were greater in Standard than in Rostral patients in respect of: decrease in suggestibility, decrease in disposition rigidity, decrease in self-criticism and smoother work curves.

On two scores Rostrals showed greater changes than Standards, viz. the improvement in the best score in manual dexterity and the speed of writing.

On traits related to introversion-extraversion the following changes were greater in Standard than in Rostral patients: increased appreciation of sex humour, increased orientation to present and future, increase in extent and intensity of self-blame, loss in endurance and differential loss in verbal and performance I.Q.

Only on one variable were changes greater in Rostral than in Standard patients. The Rostrals increased in speed more than did the Standards. This was the case with regard to the total time taken over the mazes, the total time taken over the Wechsler Arithmetic sub-test and the time on the Track Tracer trials. These results, however, should be considered in combination with those to be reported on 'accuracy'.

The patients made more mistakes on the Track Tracer after the operations. This was, however, less evident in Rostral than in Standard patients. The same was true with regard to the number of failures made on Porteus Mazes, and this was the general tendency observed on other tests not included in the above; the decrease in accuracy was *less* pronounced in Rostrals than in Standards.

It was clear with regard to the mazes, in which a failure necessitates doing the whole maze anew, that the number of failures determined in part the total time taken. The same effect of mistakes on speed is true on the Track Tracer, where making a mistake means going into a hole from which you have to come out. It follows that the Rostral patients who make fewer failures should also take less time.

A possible explanation, therefore, of the greater increase in speed shown by the Rostrals in comparison with the Standards is that this speed is partly due to the decreased accuracy being less marked in these patients. There is some additional evidence in favour of the explanation put forward. The ratio of speed to accuracy on the Track Tracer trials was calculated; it decreased after both the Standard and Rostral operations but was greater in the Standard operation.

Another difference between Rostrals and Standards may be explained in the same way. In the previous section we reported that the best trial on the Track Tracer showed a greater increase in speed after the Rostral operation than after the Standard. This result may be due to the Rostral patient making fewer mistakes than the Standard on his 'best trial' and therefore managing to do it more quickly.

Thus on traits associated with diminished introversion greater changes in scores occurred after the posterior Standard than after the anterior Rostral operation; this was true both three months and nine months after the Standard operation. On traits related to neuroticism there was a suggestion that the extent of changes following on the Standard operation was greater. The change found in intellectual aspects after the posterior operation was not present after the anterior with the exception of two items (social attitudes and reversed digits) on which it was less pronounced.

The similarity in pattern of orectic personality test changes after the posterior and anterior operations respectively has been pointed out. In order to express in quantitative terms the relationship between the two types of incision, correlations were run between the critical ratios of the differences in test scores following on the two operations. Two correlation coefficients were calculated in comparing the changes after the anterior operation with those after the posterior operation at the first follow-up, the intellectual being separated from the non-intellectual scores. The correlation coefficient between critical ratios of the Standard posterior operation at three months and the Rostral anterior operation at six months on nineteen intellectual measures was −0·400, and on thirty-two orectic personality tests it was +0·211. It will be seen that there is a marked difference on intellectual measures, while there is considerable similarity on tests of temperament and character.

A comparison of the effects of the Rostral anterior operation with that of the posterior Standard operation at the second follow-up gave a correlation coefficient for nineteen intellectual measures of −0·143 and for forty-one tests of temperament and character +0·369. After the longer period it will be seen that the changes in temperament and character tests have become increasingly similar in the two operations; while the differences on intelligence tests have decreased although there was still a negative correlation.[1] The two operations, therefore, have very similar effects on orectic aspects of personality and dissimilar effects on intellectual aspects, the posterior operation causing the deficit in the latter (Petrie, 1951).

The extent of the change in orectic traits was less in the anterior group than in the posterior group. The suggestion might be made that the loss on intellectual tests in posterior patients is partly due to the pronounced changes in their personality and that the absence of such loss in Rostral patients is to be explained in part by the less pronounced change in their personality. It might be pointed out, for example, that a change in that aspect of character involving social attitudes affects scores on the Comprehension sub-test on the Wechsler scale of intelligence and that the Standard patients' lower scores on the Comprehension sub-test is the main contributor to their loss in verbal I.Q. and the full-scale I.Q.

The change in temperament is also likely to alter behaviour on Porteus Mazes in a manner which leads to a lower I.Q. score. If a mistake is made on any maze the I.Q. score is less whether the error was made through impulsiveness or through lack of 'planning capacity'. A patient who tends to start off more quickly and to pause less on the way is likely to make more impulsive mistakes; this happened on other tests with Standard patients. By the same argument, if the Rostral patient is less impulsive and has changed less in the direction of a decrease in

[1] When both the orectic and intelligence test changes are combined in one correlation the similarities and differences between the two operations are hidden because they tend to cancel each other out. Thus at the first retest for fifty-one measurements the correlation between the Standard and Rostral operations is −0·053; at the second retest for sixty measurements it is +0·224. It follows, therefore, that such treatment of the figures is misleading.

accuracy, then his behaviour on Porteus Mazes may not be penalised to the same degree as it would have been in Standard patients.

This argument might be extended to cover at least one aspect of the change in language found in Standard patients and not in Rostral patients. It might be argued that this is due to the greater carelessness of these patients; they do not persevere and search for the right word and are less critical about the word that comes easily to mind. The less critical use of language is an example of their greater satisfaction with their own production —irrespective of its real worth—which has been noted on other tests. In the case of the proverbs, it could also be argued that with greater care a better production would be forthcoming and that many of the explanations given might be classed as 'excessively careless'.

It might even be suggested that if a series of graduated incisions were carried out ranging between the posterior Standard and anterior Rostral in position, a difference would be found in the extent of intellectual changes comparable to the extent of personality changes. But if this were the case it would be a remarkable coincidence that the anterior operation should just happen to be at that point where intellectual loss ceases to be shown. It is more likely that we have here an indication of cerebral localisation with respect to certain aspects of intelligence. The evidence would appear to point to the more posterior part of the frontal lobe playing a part in intellectual behaviour: in some way contributing to the will and ability to enlarge the area of meaning of a proverb, to the understanding and acceptance of standards of social behaviour and the will to find the right word or the capacity to recognise it when found.

It is, of course, possible that this allusive and almost irrelevant use of language is a very mild form of aphasia and that we have in some way interfered with the language centres in the posterior operation and not in the anterior operation. It would have been of interest to compare left and right unilateral *posterior* operation with regard to this particular finding. We might expect to find that if a *posterior* unilateral operation were carried out, the language difficulty would only be manifested by right-handed patients operated on the left side—but this is a matter for further research. A tendency was noticed for left dominance in right-handed people in the Rostral operation on the measures of personality, but as the language difficulties did not show themselves after any of the anterior operations we could make no deductions as to the side involved.

It is clear that it is of great advantage to the patient, when therapeutically permissible, to have a more anterior operation seeing that it does not cause the intellectual changes consequent on the posterior Standard operation. A comparison of the clinical success of the two operations is made later in this chapter.

The comparison of the results of posterior Standard and anterior Rostral leucotomy has shown that the more posterior the incision the greater the personality change; it also suggests the localisation of certain intellectual functions in the more posterior part of the frontal lobe. A study of left and right anterior operations has also suggested some localisation in the left frontal lobes of the personality changes found after leucotomy operations. It may be that this latter finding links up with the concept of left cerebral dominance in other fields.

A COMPARISON OF THE VARIATION IN THE EFFECTS OF THE OPEN ANTERIOR ROSTRAL OPERATION AND THE BLIND POSTERIOR STANDARD OPERATION

It has been mentioned that when the neurosurgeon carries out the Standard operation, he does not open up the skull of the patient to ascertain the exact location of the various parts of the frontal lobe. In the Rostral operation, on the other hand, the skull is partially opened. Professor Meyer and his associates have shown that there is considerable variation in the incisions made in a Standard operation and have suggested that the open Rostral operation leads to more precise incisions (Meyer and Beck, 1945; McLardy and Meyer, 1949; Meyer, 1950). It has been shown that part of the variability in the position of the incision is due to the elasticity of the brain tissue and part to haemorrhage and interference with blood supply. These last two factors are also present in the Rostral technique, but in a more controllable form, because it is an open operation.

A comparison of scores was made to ascertain whether the closed procedure led to more variation in the objectively measurable effects than did the open operation. After both types of operation the differences in scores on tests and the standard deviation of these differences were calculated.

The standard deviation of the difference in tests on which significant changes were found after both types of operation were compared. (The intellectual scores were not compared, as there was no loss on these in the Rostral patients such as had been found in the Standard patients.) On the four test scores related to decreased neuroticism—the standard deviation—the measure of variability was greater in the closed operation in two of the tests and greater in the open operation on two of the tests. Thus the standard deviation of the difference in self-criticism and speed of writing was much greater in the closed than in the open operation. The standard deviation of suggestibility and the highest score on the Track Tracer was slightly larger in the open operation.

On tests related to extroversion somewhat different results were found. The closed operation showed greater variability in its effects than did the open operation on all four measures related to the self-blame inventory, on both tests of perseveration, in physical endurance and in the ratio of speed to accuracy. (The greater variability in the effect of the closed operation did not manifest itself when speed was considered independently of accuracy.) The two 'miscellaneous' test changes indicating increased distractibility and an increased rate of willed fluctuation showed the same tendency. There was greater variation in the effect of the closed operation than the open. The effect of the closed Standard posterior operation, therefore, shows more variation than the open Rostral on all but one of the measures related to diminished introversion as well as on other personality tests.

In comparing the variation of the Standard with the Rostral operation we have considered both the difference found at three months and at nine months. Greater variability was found in the closed operation after the shorter as well as the longer interval with the exception of ratio of speed to accuracy.[1]

It could be argued, of course, that some of the increased variation after a Standard closed operation is due to its being

[1] Some of the tests were analysed by means of a comparison of the percentages found before and after the operation, and in such calculation the standard deviation was not included. Among these were attitude to time, appreciation of sex humour and attitude to illness. The variability in the effect of the two operations in the case of these tests has, therefore, not been calculated.

more posterior than the Rostral and that after an open posterior operation there might be greater variation than after an open anterior operation. It seems reasonable to suggest, however, that the greater variation in the effect of the blind operation must be partly, if not wholly, due to the nature of the operation rather than to the position of the incision. It appears, therefore, that there is considerable evidence from these objective tests that the open operation leads to greater precision in its effects than the blind operation.

A COMPARISON OF THE CLINICAL SUCCESS OF POSTERIOR STANDARD AND ANTERIOR ROSTRAL LEUCOTOMY

The physician in charge assessed the clinical success of the operation on each of the patients, using a five-point scale. This was an estimate of the general overall improvement of each patient, considering his pre-operative illness, his social adaptation in so far as it was known to the physician, his present symptoms and his ability to carry on without further help from the hospital. The physician was supplied with an assessment sheet for each patient and was asked to decide whether the patient was greatly improved (5), much improved (4), improved (3), unchanged (2), worse (1). It was decided to use 'improved' as the middle category after a pilot survey in which it became clear that very few patients were likely to be rated as 'worse'. (If 'unchanged' had been rated as (3) the lowest category would have been virtually unused.)

The estimate of the clinical success of the Standard approach was made approximately nine months after the operation; the estimate of the success of the Rostral operation was made a little earlier, approximately six months after the operation. The clinical ratings of twenty-seven anterior Rostral patients were compared with twenty-seven posterior Standard patients.

The numbers and percentages in each of the five categories were as follows:

	Greatly improved	Much improved	Improved	Same	Worse
Posterior Standard operation	11 (41%)	6 (22%)	4 (15%)	5 (18%)	1 (4%)
Anterior Rostral operation	0 (0%)	11 (41%)	11 (41%)	5 (18%)	0 (0%)

The striking difference between the two operations is found in the category assessed as 'greatly improved', nearly half our patients falling into this category after the posterior Standard operation and none after the anterior Rostral. On the other hand, after the anterior Rostral operation some improvement is found in twenty-two (82%) of the patients. It will also be noted that there is one patient who is worse after the posterior operation and none after the anterior operation.

The one patient who was rated 'worse' was a man of high intelligence with a responsible, creative job before he came into the hospital which he could not retain after the operation. The posterior operation may have deprived him of more than he could afford to lose if he was to carry on at his previous level of activity.

The figures of the clinical success of the operations, combined with the results on objective tests that we have reported earlier, strongly suggest that the amount of change resulting from an anterior Rostral operation is too little for some patients, though it suffices for many of them. The Standard operation, on the other hand, characterised by its more extensive destruction of tissue, is certainly causing pronounced changes in both personality and intellectual behaviour, and may be too much for some of the patients. Probably an operation midway between these two incisions, possibly slightly nearer to the Standard in position, would meet the requirements of many neurotic patients. It would appear necessary to decide on the basis of the life history and the activities of the patient as to whether a more posterior or more anterior incision will best meet his needs.

The Relationship between Successful Standard Leucotomy and Pre-operative Personality Scores

The relationship between pre-operative personality scores and improvement after the Standard operation, as estimated by the physicians in charge of each case, was examined. The rating of the improvement of each patient was made on a five-point scale and was based on the condition of the patient not earlier than nine months after the Standard operation, although in many cases the patients had been followed up from two to three years. The rating of twenty-seven patients was correlated with the pre-operative personality test scores. (The tests and scoring methods are described in Appendix A.)

There were three significant correlations. The first was the total amount of changes shown in a test of concentration; that is, the smoother the output of the patient during the eight trials on the test of concentration, the more successful was the operation ($r = -0.529$). The second concerned the goal the patients set themselves in the test of level of Aspiration. The discrepancy between the actual performance of the patients and the goals they set themselves in terms of the speed at which they proposed to do the task was calculated for the eight trials. The smaller this goal discrepancy in the patient prior to the operation, the more successful was the operation ($r = -0.397$).

The third correlation was found with regard to the ratio of speed to accuracy on the second trial on the Track Tracer. This value was high if the patient was very slow and very accurate; it was lower if the patient was making some mistakes and was working faster. The successful patient had a low speed–accuracy ratio ($r = 0.394$) prior to the operation.

All these correlations between the criterion and test scores were negative. Thus an individual who, prior to leucotomy, did not set his goal too high, had a smoother curve of concentration, was not too slow and accurate in the test of manual dexterity—in comparison with the rest of the patients—was likely to be a successful candidate for leucotomy.

It will be noted that all the significant correlations are related to tests of orectic aspects of personality and not to intelligence. All the correlations between tests of intelligence and the success of the operation were of a negligible degree. Thus, within the intelligence range of our group, the intelligence level of the patient was not related to the clinical success of the operation.

There does, however, appear to be a relationship between the patients' scores on tests related to introversion and the success of the operation. In addition to goal discrepancy and the speed–accuracy ratio we found a negative relationship—but below the level of significance—on some of the other tests associated with introversion. Thus, the speed at which the eight trials on the Track Tracer were carried out was related to success ($r = -0.243$); and on the self-blame inventory the more successful patients expressed less excessive self-blame than did the other patients ($r = 0.331$). It would seem therefore that the patients whose scores on these tests were less introverted before the operation were likely to benefit as a result of leucotomy.

The Relationship between Successful Leucotomy and the Amount of Change on Tests of Personality after the Operation

The rating of the clinical success of the operation was correlated with the amount of change on personality test scores found after the Standard operation. The differences on twenty patients between the pre-operative test scores and those at nine months' retest were used for this purpose.

On tests related to the dimension of extraversion-introversion there was one significant correlation between post-operative personality change and the estimated clinical success —the ratio of speed to mistakes on the Track Tracer ($r = 0.473$). This figure suggests that, as might have been expected, the greatest decrease in accuracy is found in the least successful patients.

Three significant correlations were found between changes on 'miscellaneous tests' of personality and a successful operation.

The first concerned the number of words produced and the time spent on a task of persistence; the successful patients were not spending more time or being more productive ($r = 0.514$ and $r = 0.622$).

The second concerned the total change in output in the series of trials in the test of concentration. There had been no noticeable trend in this score after the operation; but it appears that the successful group showed a *less* smooth curve of concentration ($r = 0.544$).

The third was the work curve on the Track Tracer which had tended to be flatter after the operation, though the change did not reach the level of significance; it appears that the flatter curve, i.e. the absence of improvement during the series of trials, was found, as might be expected, in the less successful patients ($r = 0.430$).

A number of intellectual measures showed correlations that are of interest. In each case it was found that those patients assessed by the physicians as least improved clinically showed the greatest loss on intelligence tests. Thus verbal I.Q. had dropped for the group as a whole, but the drop was greatest in our least successful patients ($r = 0·446$).

On various other intelligence scores the greatest loss was found among the least successful patients, although the correlation did not reach the level of significance; these were the full-scale Wechsler I.Q. ($r = 0·405$), the Comprehension sub-test of the Wechsler ($r = 0·259$) and Porteus Mazes mental age ($r = 0·193$).

After the Standard operation there were two suggestive increases in scores on Wechsler sub-tests. One of these was the Digit Symbol sub-test, in which symbols are substituted for a series of numbers as quickly as possible. The greatest improvement on this sub-test was found on our successful patients ($r = 0·528$). The other score showing an increase was memory for digits as measured by the difference between those in the order given and those remembered in reversed order. The patients had shown a tendency for this difference to increase after the operation; the correlation indicated that the difference was greatest in the most successful patients ($r = 0·490$). On all measures of intelligence our successful patients lost least, or even gained, as opposed to our unsuccessful patients.

Those patients who, *before* the operation, on personality tests showed low goals, low ratio of speed to mistakes in the test of manual dexterity and had a smoother concentration work-curve appeared to be most successful clinically. On these three scores the successful patients showed *less* change after the operation than did the unsuccessful patients. As there appeared to be a strong tendency for this to happen on many of the other tests, a correlation was run between these two sets of correlations; that is, between those of pre-operative personality and success and those of post-operative changes and success. The size of the resultant coefficient was $-0·479$. There appears, therefore, to be a significant negative relationship between pre-operative personality and the post-operative changes in so far as these are related to a successful operation.

The significant correlations reported above indicate a relationship between the amount of a certain score and the success of the operation. It should be pointed out, however, that the correlation may be curvilinear or rectilinear; if the former, it means that loss (or gain) beyond a certain point is disadvantageous to these patients. As the numbers of patients are not large enough to determine the exact nature of the correlation, the question of the exact relationship must be left open. It is possible, however, that with regard to all the correlations which have been reported a certain amount of change is advantageous from the clinical viewpoint but that change beyond that amount is undesirable. It may be true, for example, that in certain patients some change in intellectual functioning is necessary for a clinically adjudged success but that the point of 'diminishing returns' is soon reached. This may also be the case with regard to pre-operative scores.

It will be remembered that the Rostral operation was less successful clinically than the Standard. The main differences were that in the effect on personality of the Rostral operation there was no loss on intelligence tests and the extent of the change on the orectic personality tests was smaller. It is probable that these characteristics of the Rostral operation are contributory to its being less successful. As far as intelligence is concerned this may mean that a slight loss is necessary in leucotomy patients, but that the amount of the loss after the Standard operation was too great. There may be an opportunity of confirming this hypothesis from the results of using an operation midway between the Standard and Rostral in position and finding what effect it has clinically and on these personality tests.

Having reported on the ways in which we have used the clinical assessments of improvement, it is necessary to make certain reservations regarding these results. In the original plan for the criterion of improvement it had been intended to include an assessment by the employer of the patient in so far as his ability at his work was concerned, an assessment by the relatives in so far as ability to live with the family was concerned[1] and it was also proposed to obtain an assessment by the patient himself of his condition. We had hoped to use these different assessments to obtain a total picture of the patient's condition. In fact, through circumstances beyond our control, we have been able to obtain only the clinical assessments for all the

[1] Since writing the above, a piece of work has been completed by Dr. Macdonald Tow, one of the chief features of which was the interviewing of patients' relatives before and after leucotomy (Tow, 1951).

patients. Clearly although this assessment is the most reliable of the four to use on its own, it is not as reliable as would have been a suitably weighted combination of four separate judgments. These results, therefore, and their interpretation are put forward with somewhat more reserve than other clearly defined trends reported in this chapter.

CHAPTER SIX

SYNTHESIS AND CONCLUSIONS

THE conclusions which emerge from the investigations reported in the rest of the book will be discussed and some of their implications considered in this chapter. With certain reservations the broad statement can be made that the use of objective tests of personality before and after leucotomy enables us to predict the constellation of personality changes following on different types of frontal lobe operations. The pattern of personality changes has been shown to be consistent in the four different types of operation examined, and the alteration in traits may be readily grouped so as to demonstrate changes in the dimensions of personality—viz. a decrease in the strength of traits associated with neuroticism and with intro-version and a decrease in certain aspects of intelligence, as shown in the Summary Table.[1] The tests also enable us to take count of the differences in the effect of these operations. Altera-tions in personality are more pronounced after the posterior Standard operation than the anterior Rostral operation, par-ticularly as shown in the table in the sphere of intelligence; and unilateral left operations appear to contribute more than do those on the right to the effect of bilateral Rostral leucotomy.

The changes which follow the Standard operation—after both the shorter and longer interval—the Rostral operation, and the differences between the two allow of remarkably clear-cut deductions, though in view of the small number of patients the differences in the effect of right and left operations are put for-ward with more reserve. The differences observed are probably significant, but more extensive research would be required to put them on a firm foundation. Doubt and uncertainty surround the data which did not attain the required standard of statistical significance—a fact which has been mentioned on each occasion.

[1] See page 98.

Some hesitancy has been felt in reporting on prognostic indicators and the relationship between the amount of change following on the operation and the success of the operation. Such a relationship has only been reported when it has reached the level of significance, but it is felt that there is considerable room for improvement in the selection of suitable criteria for judging post-operative success. This might be attained by increasing the number of clinical judges and by enlarging the area in which success is estimated to include the opinions regarding the patient of his medical advisers, family and employers.

We are not suggesting that the effect of an incision in the frontal lobes provides us at the same time with the knowledge of all the functions of this part of the brain. It could not be claimed, for example, that because the loss of both eyes leads to blindness, the function of eyes is to prevent blindness. But just as the study of blindness enables us to understand, if not the nature, the advantages of sight, so the study of defects following on frontal lobe operations may enable us to understand the advantage of possessing them in an intact condition.

We feel fairly confident that the picture a patient presents after leucotomy is likely to correspond closely to that of an individual with obliterative lesions in this part of the brain. Part of this confidence is due to the type of patient who formed the basis of this investigation, namely, neurotics with well-preserved personalities.[1] Investigators in the past, studying the effect of traumatic injury to the frontal lobe, have usually done so on chronic psychotics and have been confronted with the difficulty of estimating the previous personality of these psychotics. An attempt was made to estimate 'the glory that was Greece and the grandeur that was Rome' before the ruin set in, but it remained a guess, and a hazardous one at that.

The present investigation was planned on the traits associated with two of the personality dimensions in a neurotic population, which has been shown to be quite distinct from the dimensions in a psychotic population (Eysenck, 1950). Absence of identity

---

[1] It will be noted from the diagnostic categories that most of the patients were neurotics. Although a few might have been otherwise classified by different psychiatrists this would not alter the main import of the conclusions on the seventy patients discussed in this book.

SUMMARY TABLE

CHANGES AFTER THE TWO TYPES OF OPERATION

(Changes in direction predicted by hypotheses in italic)

* Change less pronounced in Rostral than in Standard patients.

† Only found at 3 months

	Changes in personality after posterior Standard bilateral leucotomy (closed operation)	Changes in personality after anterior Rostral bilateral leucotomy (open operation)
TRAITS RELATED TO NEUROTICISM		
Suggestibility	*Decreased*	*Decreased**
Disposition rigidity	*Lower Perseveration scores*	*Lower perseveration scores**
Manual dexterity (best score of series of eight)	*Improvement*	*Improvement*
Speed of writing	*Increased*	*Increased*
Self-criticism	*Decreased*	*Decreased**
Speed on mental and manual tasks	*Increased*	*Increased*
TRAITS RELATED TO INTROVERSION		
Accuracy on mental and manual tasks	*Decreased*	Suggestive change—decreased
Self-blame (in relation to personality characteristics)		
Extent of self-blame	*Decreased*	*Decreased**
Intensity of self-blame	*Decreased*	*Decreased**
Self-blame (in relation to failure at an insoluble task)	*Decreased*	*Decreased**

	Attitude to past, present and future	Increased orientation to present as opposed to past	Increased orientation to present as opposed to past*
	Liking for sex humour	Increased	Increased*
	Ratio of verbal to performance intelligence scores	Decreased	Decreased*
MISCELLANEOUS PERSONALITY TESTS	Endurance	Decreased	Suggestive decrease
	Control of fluctuation of ambiguous figure	Increased	Increased*
	Concentration	Suggestive change — improved	Improved
	Estimation of time	Suggestive change—time passes more quickly	Time passes more quickly
	Distractibility	Suggestive change — increased	Suggestive change — increased
INTELLECTUAL TESTS	Wechsler total I.Q.	Decreased	No change
	Wechsler verbal I.Q.	Decreased	No change
	Social comprehension test	Decreased	No change
	Performance I.Q.	No change	No change
	Porteus Mazes I.Q.	Decreased†	No change
	Generalisation in interpretation of proverbs	Decreased	No change
	Misuse of language	Increased	No change
	Style of writing and content of written material	Changed	Changed*
VARIATION IN PERSONALITY CHANGES	Social attitudes	Changed	Changed*
	Orectic personality tests	Greater	Smaller

of the dimensions amongst neurotic and psychotic populations apart, it is not surprising that for other reasons psychotics do not show clear-cut changes. As Mettler (1950) points out, disabilities of the type reported to result from leucotomy are exceedingly difficult to detect in psychotic patients. Schizophrenics, for example, are not entirely cured of their schizophrenia, if indeed it is at all improved by the operation. In a schizophrenic one is studying the effect of the operation on individuals already permanently altered by an illness which is inextricably interwoven with the effect of the latter on personality. The greater that illness the less clearly will be shown the changes in personality due to the operation alone.

Mettler (1950) suggests that defects in higher functioning resulting from operating on the frontal lobes might not appear for other reasons. He mentions that there is abundant evidence indicating that physiological defects produce varying effects in individuals of essentially different personality. Where the basic personality differed to the extent that a psychoneurotic does from an institutionalised deteriorated schizophrenic, one would not expect that leucotomy would produce identical reactions in both. In addition to the effect of the psychosis on personality pattern both before and after the operation, there is a considerable difference in these two populations in testability, cooperativeness and rapport with the examiner. Hence the absence of defect in psychotics after leucotomy is but suggestive evidence at the best regarding the effect of frontal lobe lesions in non-psychotics. Nevertheless, the apparent absence of deficit may be regarded as a justification for undertaking the operation in psychotics with little fear of harming them more than their psychoses have already done.

Our patients were, however, severe neurotics. An ideal estimate of the effect of frontal lobe lesion would be obtained from the results of the operation on completely normal individuals. As this is clearly not possible, we must be content with the results obtained on those who are most nearly normal of those operated on. It is on such that the present report is made.

The difference between performance before and after the operation has been the basis of these results. It will be apparent that had the scores after the operation been considered on their own they would have told us nothing. The practice, which is by no means uncommon, of taking patients after leucotomy and contrasting them with a so-called comparable group who have not undergone the operation is somewhat unfortunate. Some of the disappointments in the contribution of psychological methods to understanding the effects of leucotomy have resulted from this practice.

The operation was performed with a view to alleviating the neurotic condition of the patients. Most of them were much better after the operation; that is, their neurotic symptoms had subsided. It might be argued that the changes we have found do not result from the operation itself but from alleviation of the mental illness which the operation has produced. This argument could indeed hold for the change in measurements associated with neuroticism. We would expect that the decrease in neuroticism resulting from the operation might lead to changes which differentiate the extreme neurotic from the less neurotic, which we have listed earlier. The decline in neuroticism would not, however, account for the changes after leucotomy on trait measurements associated with the dimension of extraversion-introversion, as no such relationship appeared in the numerous investigations on these tests which have been carried out.

Moreover, it would certainly be difficult to extend an explanation based on alleviation of illness to cover the changes found in verbal ability, social comprehension, the use of language, planning and so on. Had these improved, one might have suspected that the illness prior to the operation had interfered with performance. But the loss we have found demands explanation by reference to the functions of an intact frontal lobe.

In trying to estimate the effect of a lesion in a particular position in the frontal lobe, we have had the advantage of seeing patients all of whom have been operated upon by the same neurosurgeon, Mr. Wylie McKissock, who enjoys a unique experience in this field. Although of necessity there occurs some variation in the position of the incision, the lesions produced by one surgeon differ from each other much less than do those produced by different surgeons. Moreover, whilst in closed operations incisions based on cranial landmarks do not invariably involve identical regions, in the open Rostral operation one can be more certain that this was the case.

In trying to understand personality changes following on prefrontal leucotomy, Flugel (1949), amongst others, has stressed the need to examine the measurements associated with the factors of personality that have so far been identified. This has been done in the present investigation. The tests chosen have primarily been those already shown to be related to neuroticism and to introversion and extraversion. This has been found to be a profitable approach in delineating the broad tendencies that result from each type of operation, as well as the changes in the individual personality traits that characterise the leucotomy patient. Although some interesting differences became apparent in using purely intellectual measures, such understanding as we have been able to obtain of the effect of incisions in the frontal lobe is based on a consideration of measures of temperament, character and intelligence in combination.

We do not know how much the change of temperament is related to the change in intellectual activity. Yet we may be permitted to recall the time when scientists had difficulty in accepting the concept that mass alters with velocity. Have we perhaps now arrived at the point where the social and medical sciences will need to consider the possibility that intelligence alters with temperament?

An attempt has been made throughout to use tests which can be repeated in an identical form by other investigators, and where the scoring is objective. It might be argued that our use of questionnaires and subjective information from the patient did not conform with this standard. Such criticism would have been justified had this subjective information been regarded as being a true account of the patient's personality; in fact our use of such data has always been on the basis of 'this is what the patient says about himself.' For example, in pointing out the traits on which patients regarded themselves as changed after leucotomy it was stressed that this was a self-portrait by an individual who was not over-blessed with insight and had an exalted opinion of himself; but it was nevertheless a self-portrait. It is in this sense that the data from questionnaires have been used.

Having obtained measurements of changes in personality we have leaned heavily on statistical analysis to sort the wheat from the chaff. An attempt has been made not to overburden the reader with statistical detail, but this does not mean that useful results could have been reported without such an analysis. As Cattell (1950) has said, 'Statistical analysis is a device to bring out relationships and patterns which unaided observation and memory could not perceive. It does for the mind, struggling in an unfocussed chaos of facts, what the microscope does for the unaided eye.'

Changes in personality traits have been reported in the form 'the patients became more inaccurate'; 'they were quicker after the operation'. This, of course, means that in the comparison with their behaviour before the operation, whatever that may have been, they made more mistakes or were quicker. It should be remembered, however, that there was great variation in behaviour before leucotomy. The characteristic of the group as a whole was the change in the same direction on all the variables. It is also necessary to emphasise that the terms used to describe these tests and the changes they measure must not be interpreted in the popular sense. They refer to direct quantitative variables and the findings should not be enlarged beyond this limitation.

This does not mean that the investigations carried out under laboratory conditions are irrelevant to behaviour in everyday life. Such an argument was used at the beginning of this century about intelligence tests, when it was thought that a sampling of behaviour in such an artificial situation could not contribute to one's knowledge of a man's innate ability. It has now become clear that the contribution made by such tests is dependent on the adequacy of the sample of his mental activity. At the time of writing too many people tend to believe that, in the intellectual sphere, all questions can be answered about an individual after three-quarters of an hour of intelligence testing. The truth lies somewhere between these two extremes. A great deal that is relevant to an individual's everyday behaviour can be ascertained if investigations into all aspects of personality are carried out—temperament, character and intelligence.

In each investigation patients were seen for a total of approximately six hours. During this time, in addition to performance on the tests selected, there were opportunities to observe the patients' reactions to different occurrences and to listen to their comments. It is extremely unlikely that for a period of this length an artificial 'act' was being maintained. The impression gained from these interviews accentuated the picture obtained from objective test scores.

It should be observed that there was some indication that the patients' reaction to stress was less marked after than before the operation, and also that unpleasant tasks were less disliked. For example, a patient, in talking of herself, said she didn't mind things going wrong any more; that an ambulance had driven up to her house the previous day and that she hadn't been in the least concerned. She was quite sure that before leucotomy she would have been in a shocking state wondering what had happened and to whom. Another patient volunteered, 'It changed me. I don't want to work so hard at home.' Still another, when a letter was handed to me whilst she was in the room, volunteered, 'I don't like writing letters any more; I like receiving them and not answering them.'

Many reports of post-leucotomy patients suggest that they are more tactless and more abrupt in their manners after the operation (Freeman and Watts, 1942; Partridge, 1950). A possible explanation of the cause of this increased insensitivity to the feelings of others is based on the changes we have found in the patients in this investigation. They are less self-critical, less concerned about their fate and achievements, and less concerned about social standards. Their vulnerability to the 'slings and arrows of outrageous fortune' has decreased. It may be that in this way they have lost the use of the barometer they previously had to gauge the climate of the reactions of others. The subtleties of human relationship—of what is painful and what is permissible—are constantly being impressed on us by our own experience in society. Being tactful is a much more complex form of behaviour than not hurting another person in the physical sense. It would be possible to argue that a man who loses his sense of physical pain would nevertheless remember what type of things caused pain to others; and therefore would not inflict a great deal of physical damage on the people round him. This has been shown to be the case in the rare patient who has complete loss of painful sensation with general paralysis of the insane. But the infliction of psychic pain depends on so many variables that we are constantly relearning the rules in our own relationship with the people round us. Perhaps leucotomy patients have difficulty for the reason suggested—their own decreased vulnerability to psychic pain—in relearning these rules.

In this connection it is necessary to remember that psychic pain may be important in many different ways to man. To take an analogy involving physical pain, it is pertinent to consider one of the rare cases of a child born without any sensation of pain (Boyd and Niel, 1949). This child would bite her own tongue so that it became scarred and jagged; she would sit on the fire and would be rescued by her family because they would smell the scent of burning flesh; a broken limb would be unnoticed and the continued use would do it further damage. In the absence of the protective mechanism of pain, every effort made by the environment to protect this child was inadequate. Moreover, this child unwittingly but continually inflicted physical damage on her friends because she could not visualise this particular effect of her action. This underlines the fundamental biological function of pain. No attempt will be made to explore the complex area of the usefulness of psychic pain and the manner in which it may act as a warning of threats to the personality: but there is every reason to believe that the patient after leucotomy is less sensitive to psychic pain than he was before the operation.[1]

It is also of interest that Brain (1951) attaches so much importance to the part which emotion and imagery play in human achievement because emotion provides the motive power which sustains our course of action, and if action is to take time the object to which it is directed must be constantly represented to us by means of mental imagery. Our results suggest that a leucotomy patient has diminished emotion and there is also some evidence to suggest that he has less vivid mental imagery.

It is hoped that by delaying the second examination to nine

[1] Of interest in this connection are the experimental studies with monkeys (Freudenberg *et al.*, 1950), particularly the 'loss of sense of danger' in monkeys after lesions in the cingular gyrus and adjacent areas described by Glees *et al.* (1950). The authors suggest that in the jungle stage this deficiency would not be consistent with survival.

months after the operation sufficient time has been allowed for the results to indicate the more permanent state of the patient and not just a temporary phase. The close relationship between the results we have obtained after intervals of three months and nine months makes it clear that this is not a temporary state, due to the trauma of the operation. On the other hand, the longer one waits the more likely it is that one is witnessing an adaptation to the original deficit. As Mettler (1949) has said, 'Only rarely can one observe a physiological deficit directly; more usually what one sees is the organism's compensatory behaviour in the presence of such a deficit.' The fact that some of the changes are more evident after the longer period does perhaps suggest that we are witnessing an increasingly adequate adaptation. The ingenuity with which compensations for lost functions are made by the body is well known to clinicians. Guttman (1946) has shown to what lengths this can go when he has trained airmen with severed spinal cords to control their leg movements by means of muscles running from the shoulders. But such evidence as we have suggests that the adaptability of the brain surpasses that of the rest of the body; indeed, as Hughlings Jackson (1890) pointed out, any suggestion of cerebral localisation really means that this is a preferred area for fulfilling a certain function, but that such function can at any time—and almost as conveniently—be taken over by some other part of the brain.

Does this suggest that the effects we have found after incisions on the frontal lobe are not peculiar to this area and might be found with lesions of any other part of the hemisphere? There are many reports in the literature of the differential effect of lesions of various parts of the hemisphere (Rylander, 1943; Alcade, 1947; Yahn, 1949). To mention details of just one: a careful study has been carried out of the pattern of differences in frontal lesions and parietal lesions and it was found that whilst the parietal group resembles anxiety neurotics, the frontal group resembles the hysteric (extraverted type) which we have described here (Anderson and Hanvic, 1950). Moreover, the results here reported, showing that there are clear-cut differences according to which part of the frontal lobe is affected by the incision, suggest that there are special functions which are interfered with in leucotomy of various types and that these functions are different from those involved in other cerebral operations. This, however, will require further research.

It has been shown, however, that in leucotomy, when the connections between parts of the frontal areas and the rest of the brain are severed, and in topectomy, where an area of the frontal cortex is removed, the effects resulting are the same (Mettler, 1949).

SPECULATIVE POSSIBILITIES

The Success of the Operation of Leucotomy in the Relief of Intractable Pain

Although none of the operations reported here were done purely for the relief of intractable pain, our results may throw some light on how incisions in the frontal lobes achieve this result. It has been suggested that the change in attitude to intractable pain is closely bound up with the change in personality following on leucotomy, in that patients who remain unrelieved of pain show little personality change, whilst the contrary is true of those who are relieved (Krayenbuhl and Stoll, 1949). Many investigators have shown (Chapman *et al.*, 1948; Le Beau and Pecker, 1950) that sensitivity to painful stimuli is, if anything, greater after the operation than before. That is, the threshold of pain is, if anything, lower after leucotomy; hence the relief of intractable pain cannot be explained as being the result of greater insensitivity to painful stimuli. This relief may, however, be partly due to the change in attitude we have noted with regard to the past, present and future. After the posterior operation the range of interest in time had shrunk, being primarily concerned with the present. If, as a result of this, patients are not concerned with the pain that may be coming nor with the pain that is past, they have only the present pain to contend with. It is, of course, impossible to estimate how much the memory of past and fear of future pain contributes to the total painful state; but it is not unreasonable to suggest that if the past and future components are cut out, even partially, the total situation becomes more endurable.

It is perhaps worth noting that for most cases requiring relief of pain the more posterior operation is necessary. We found a greater change in attitude to the past and future after the posterior operation; there may be a relationship between the more outstanding changes in time attitude and the success of the particular operation.

Another of our findings appeared to be relevant to the alleviation of intractable pain. On two separate and different test-approaches time appeared to go more quickly after the operation than before; hence it is to be supposed that whatever the present represents to them as individuals, it is more quickly over; it, so to speak, becomes the past sooner than it did before the operation. This may also contribute to the decrease in preoccupation with the total painful situation.

It is also of interest in this connection to mention that it was reported that the control of fluctuation of an ambiguous figure has been shown by Gordon (1950) to be related to the control of imagery. Those who show least control in fluctuation have the most vivid imagery. The results on leucotomy patients therefore suggest that they have less vivid imagery after the operation. The perception of present pain is presumably almost inextricably interwoven with one's imagery of the pain that has gone and the pain that is to come. If the post-leucotomy patient has indeed less vivid imagery, this could also contribute to his decreased preoccupation with his own painful situation, as both anticipation and memory would be less.

One other finding seems worth mentioning in this connection; that is, the increase in distractibility we noticed after the posterior operation. This might be regarded as an advantage if the patient is suffering from intractable pain. The entertainments round him, the people's conversation, the material things that are happening in his environment will take his mind off whatever else he happened to be concentrating on. If this is his total painful situation, it will be of advantage in so far as his preoccupation with his own misfortune is concerned. Indeed, it has been shown that distracting stimuli interfere with pain judgment (Wolff and Goodell, 1943); and this finding has been independently confirmed recently (Clausen and King, 1950).

It is not suggested that the objective changes mentioned above are anything but contributory factors to the total effect. It would, however, seem desirable to explore further the impact of this type of change on attitude to a painful situation.

With regard to the lower pain threshold found in post-leucotomy patients, there is an interesting comparison to be

made between their reaction to painful stimuli and their performance on the tests of endurance that we have used in our
investigation. After Standard posterior leucotomy patients display markedly less endurance in an uncomfortable physical
situation than they did before the operation. We have suggested that this may be partly a reflection of the change in the
standards they set themselves. They see no particular reason to
endure, to persist in a painful situation. There is less compulsion
to 'grit their teeth' and bear it! In the same way we would
suggest they respond to painful stimuli earlier than they did
before the operation because they see less point in holding out.

On the other hand, after the operation the patients were
more productive and remained longer at the simple mental
task of word-building than before. It has been suggested that in
the case of mental tasks the 'tiredness' experienced by an
individual is due largely to mental conflict. If one of the results
of the operation is to reduce conflict, there should also be a
reduction in the tiredness experienced during mental tasks. This
might be noticeable on such a task as word-building, in spite of
the tendency to give up earlier after the operation. This theory,
if correct, would fit the facts as we have found them.

Social Attitudes

Golla (1946) made observations on the leucotomy patients'
impairment in the ability to make ethical evaluations. A
change in social attitude has been found in these patients both
in their written essays and in answers to questions on social
comprehension. Other suggestions emerge from the results of
the effect of leucotomy on conscience: whether we speak of it as
the 'self-regarding sentiment' of McDougall or the 'super ego'
of Freud, the behaviour of these patients indicates that it is
much less exacting after the operation. This is suggested, for
example, by the loss in endurance, the lower standards set,
greater satisfaction with self and performance, the decrease in
guilt feelings as well as in accuracy and lastly the increased
appreciation of sex humour. It is interesting that so many of the
changes we have found in patients after leucotomy fit so well
with the hypothesis that their conscience is less severe. Carelessness in the use of language has also been demonstrated; Stengel
(1937 and 1939) suggests that it is part of the function of

conscience to see to the observance of the codes that regulate the use of language.

Franz (1907) found that alteration of frontal lobes led to the loss of recently formed habits. If in man removal of these areas leads to a loss in the acceptance of social standards, may this not be due to these being a recently acquired habit? The acceptance of social standards may be habits which have to be relearned by each individual to meet the pressure of society; amongst such are those involved in accepting the desirability of being painstaking, of setting high standards and of putting up with the unendurable.

The relearning, possible in topectomised animals of recently formed 'habits', would explain the apparent social improvement in leucotomised individuals during the course of years under the continuous pressure of society which insists on the maintenance of its standards.

Social life has developed side by side with the frontal lobe; it is therefore not surprising that leucotomy should destroy some of the finer social feelings. In any case the effects consequent on leucotomy suggest that a careful study of various frontal lobe incisions and the resulting changes in social attitudes would be desirable and rewarding.

Some Considerations regarding Obsessional Patients

In relation to the changes in social attitudes discussed in the previous section, certain underlying factors need to be taken into consideration. If the loss in social attitudes happens to an individual who starts by having fairly low standards he may, as a result of his operation, be socially unacceptable. If, on the other hand, he starts by having high social standards his loss, although clearly shown both on tests and observed by the people round him, may still leave him with reasonably adequate standards of behaviour for his environment.

Psychiatrists have noticed that in comparing the population of a mental hospital with the population of a prison there is a marked absence of obsessionals in the latter (Simpson and Barnes, 1951). This suggests that obsessionals set themselves higher standards of behaviour than some of the other group of neurotics. If this is indeed the case there may be some relationship between the finding that the obsessionals are among the most successful leucotomy patients (Freeman and Watts, 1942; Partridge, 1950) and that they are found so infrequently in prison populations. Both these facts may well be due to the highly developed social attitude of the obsessional, for if an obsessional patient starts by having very high standards of social behaviour, their lowering by the operation will yet leave him sufficiently endowed to satisfy his environment. We have shown in the research reported here that there is a loss in social attitudes after prefrontal leucotomy; we have not been able to so subdivide our patients as to determine what happens to the obsessional group in comparison with other groups, seeing that the numbers in each category would not be large enough for us to make deductions of this kind. This appears to be an interesting field which invites further research.

Social Function of the Frontal Lobe

These investigations on the effect of incisions on the frontal lobes have shown that the personality alters in ways that are particularly relevant to man's relationship to society. We have found, for example, a difference in the social attitude concerned with the keeping of a promise. We have noted that after leucotomy social qualities are less frequently mentioned, whilst consideration and kindness shown direct to the patient are more often reported; that there is less feeling of personal responsibility; and that there is a strong tendency to direct criticism outwards. The patient after leucotomy is more satisfied with himself, with his capacities, with his style of living and style of writing and is less preoccupied with getting things just right; his standards have dropped.

There is also a change in the attitude to the past. The patient is much less preoccupied, interested or worried about the past. To a less extent this is also true with regard to the future. Interests, concern, happiness, thought are mainly centred in the present.

The range of time with which the individual is concerned has shrunk, so to speak, and is now more or less confined to that which is here and now. The range of interests has so far shrunk as to include little more than those who directly impinge on the patients' immediate life. The extent of the area which does so impinge varies, of course, in each individual; the important point, however, is that after the operation the area seems to have diminished.

It is relevant to consider the development of the frontal lobes in the life history of the individual. Turner (1948, 1950) has shown that both in size and in the complexity of the surface area the frontal lobes continue to develop later than the rest of the brain and that development may not cease until as late as the age of 10. There appears to be a period of intensive growth between the ages of 2 and 5.

Whilst further research into the development of the frontal lobes in children may indicate considerable individual variation, there is some ground for suggesting that the functions subserved by the frontal lobes will be found to be developing independently from and later than other broad areas of mental development.

A study, not of the child's brain but of the child's developing personality, led Freud and many others to point to the full development of conscience or super ego somewhere round the age of 5. Prior to this stage, it is suggested that the child behaves as his own impulses direct him: he has no standards of his own as to what is right or wrong and what should or should not be done. Control of his behaviour only results from the reactions of the adults around him. This control is achieved by praise or blame, reward or punishment—the chief punishment probably being the threat that love may be withdrawn. He has to live by adult standards; he has as yet none of his own. Freud explains the development of the super ego as an internalisation of the standards of behaviour which the child has seen round him, particularly in the person of his father and mother. After these standards have been internalised, the child is exceedingly strict with himself. Sometimes, it may be because of the projection of his own hostility as well as for other reasons, he makes greater demands on his own behaviour than did the people from whom he derived these standards. The family unit which received his obedience, his loyalty, his kindness and consideration is later enlarged to include gradually not only those people with whom he comes into direct contact, but society in general and perhaps, in the best of men, humanity itself.

The development of conscience and standards of behaviour is clearly a very complex process in which there is a two-way reaction between the individual and the environment. There must of necessity be infinite variation in the final product—if indeed we can speak of finality in this connection.

If there is some area of the brain concerned with this aspect of the development of human personality, the frontal lobe appears a likely place. This is suggested firstly because of what happens to a human being after a posterior leucotomy in his attitude to himself and society which we have tried to summarise above; and, secondly, because the development of the frontal lobes in the history of the child appears to be parallel to the development of his own standards of behaviour with regard to society.

It has, however, been shown that the loss in social attitudes following on this operation is relatively small and that the patient continues to be able to live fairly adequately in society afterwards. Ödegärd (1947) has suggested that the intellectual capacity of leucotomised patients is not greatly reduced because man does not use all his cortical cells and therefore has a considerable reserve to fall back on when required. We would suggest that he has perhaps a reserve for the development of ethical attitudes.

The African native can live for generations without using his brain for any problem comparable with a compound algebraic equation, a problem in solid geometry or complex arguments concerning the fourth dimension. Yet his capacities for doing all these things are present, as can be shown by his ability within one generation to do them with the proper training. He has, it appears, much greater intellectual capacity than he normally uses. Indeed, a loss in intellectual capacity which would be incapacitating in an individual living in complex Western civilisation might be almost overlooked in an untrained African native living the life of his forefathers, as there would be so few aspects of his activity which involved the capacity that he had lost.

If man's social conscience as we know it to-day demands the use of only a small part of the nervous tissues on which such attitudes depend, one might expect that the effect of operative interference with these tissues would be relatively slight. This indeed is what we have found.

APPENDIX A

DETAILED DESCRIPTION OF TESTS

DETAILED DESCRIPTION OF TECHNIQUES USED

To facilitate easy reference we are including a detailed description of the administration of each of the personality tests, the results of which have been described in Chapters II, IV and V. The order used will correspond as closely as possible to that in which the results have been reported. It is hoped that other workers will use them. But the descriptions given here, although sufficient for those desirous of following our results, cannot enable those unfamiliar with the tests to administer them. It is essential that the tests should be given in a standardised manner and this requires some special training.

Details of the Wechsler Bellevue Scale (1946) and the Porteus Mazes (1933), our two main intelligence tests, will be found in the references given, and will not be repeated here.

The six proverbs which patients were asked to explain the meaning of were as follows:

'A burnt child dreads fire.'
'He who eats the kernel must crack the nut.'
'A drowning man will catch at a straw.'
'No wind can do him good who steers for no port.'
'We only know the worth of water when the well is dry.'
'Don't judge a book by its cover.'

The same proverbs were presented before and on two occasions after the Standard operation. Samples of answers are presented in Chapter III.

TESTS RELATED TO NEUROTICISM

1. *Suggestibility. Body Sway Test and Static Ataxia*

The Body Sway test of suggestibility was introduced by Hull (1923). The subject is told to stand quite still and relax with his

114

eyes closed, and the amount of sway is measured during the period of one minute. This is the Static Ataxia score and sway without suggestion. While still in the same position, the suggestion is made to the subject that he is falling forward. It is made in the form 'you are falling forward, you are falling forward, you are falling forward all the time, you are falling, you are falling forward, you are falling forward now, you are falling forward . . .' and so on. This is continued for a period of two minutes. The amount of sway resulting from this suggestion is measured.

The measurement of sway is achieved by means of a thread which is pinned to the back of the collar of the patient, and which passes over a smooth hook and ends in a weight. The weight is in such a position that it swings up and down on a scale marked off in half-inches which is attached to the wall. The following scores resulting from this test were utilised:

1. The amount of sway occurring prior to any suggestion being made.
2. The amount of sway occurring during the period of suggestion.
3. The difference between the amount of sway occurring with and without suggestion.

2. Disposition Rigidity. Tests of Perseveration

(a) Alternation of a habitual and non-habitual activity

This test of perseveration is described by Cattell (1946B). The patient is asked to write the figures 2, 3, 4 on a sheet of lined paper as quickly as possible during a period of one minute. A demonstration is then given of writing the figures 2, 3, 4 with reversed stroke, starting each figure at the opposite end to that which is customary, 2 and 3 being written from the base upwards. The patient is given one trial to make sure that he knows what is required. He is then asked to write 2, 3, 4 with reversed stroke as quickly as possible in a period of one minute. The perseveration score is arrived at by comparing his output in the habitual activity with his output in the non-habitual activity. If he has great difficulty in the non-habitual activity, and his output is therefore much lower on this than on the habitual activity, he has a high perseveration score.

(b) A test of perseveration involving an alternation between writing a real word and a nonsense word

One form of this test was described by Cattell (1946B), who reports it as being most highly related to the factor of perseveration. The patient is asked to write the word 'ready' on lined paper as many times as possible during a period of one minute. He is then asked to write 'ydear' as frequently as possible during a period of a minute. The perseveration score is arrived at as in test (a), by comparing the output during the two periods.

3. *Manual Dexterity*

The highest score achieved in a series of trials on the Track Tracer

The Track Tracer is a machine designed in the Cambridge Laboratory and kindly loaned by Professor Bartlett. It consists of an ivorene sheet attached to a metal base. The ivorine sheet is perforated by pairs of holes which are irregularly spaced, but which define a curved path which leads from the outside of the board to the centre of the board. The patient's task is to trace the path with a stylus between these pairs of holes to the centre of the board. If he goes into a hole, electrical contact is made through the metal sheet with an electric counter and an electric buzzer. The time taken on each trial is measured on a stopwatch. We thus have a measure of both the speed and accuracy with which the patient carries out eight such trials.

The task is explained to the patient and he is asked to complete it 'as *quickly* and as *accurately*' as he can, both words being equally stressed. The trial which is done at the greatest speed is counted as the highest score. The first trial is always excluded for this purpose as constituting a practice run.

4. *Tempo of Handwriting*

The tempo of handwriting is estimated by:

(a) The number of times that the figures 2, 3, 4 can be written in a period of a minute.

(b) The number of times the word 'ready' can be written in the period of one minute.

A pencil, lined paper and a time-interval clock are used in each case.

5. *Inferiority Feelings shown in Self-rating*

The number of unpleasant traits ascribed to themselves by patients

A list of undesirable personality traits which are often ascribed to themselves by neurotics was prepared. After some preliminary experimental investigations, forty-two of these were selected. The patient is asked verbally whether he thinks he displays each of these characteristics. His answers, with the qualifications given, are noted down. The list is as follows:

1. Lazy	23. Neglectful
2. Irritable	24. Hostile
3. Impatient	25. Resentful
4. Extravagant	26. Hesitant
5. Ungrateful	27. Ungenerous
6. Excitable	28. Unjust
7. Uncontrolled	29. Unconscientious
8. Silly	30. A 'giving in' person
9. Unworthy	31. A person who doesn't 'play
10. Selfish	the game'
11. Unkind	32. Bad-tempered
12. Stingy	33. Greedy
13. A 'nagger'	34. Despondent
14. Moody	35. Over-serious
15. Unsuccessful	36. Not persistent
16. Stupid	37. Uninterested (in people)
17. Careless	38. Uninterested (in the world)
18. Dishonest	39. Shut in
19. Ambitious	40. Easily persuaded
20. Cowardly	41. Fussy
21. Unco-operative	42. A worrier
22. Talkative	

The total number of unpleasant qualities ascribed to themselves by each patient is calculated. For the purpose of estimating an increase or decrease of feelings of inferiority regarding personality, the totals before and after the operation are compared.

6. *Smoothness of Work Curve*

The smoothness of the work curve was estimated with regard to various tasks on which a series of trials was given. These included the number of figures given in a series of eight trials of concentration, the speed of tapping in four quarter-minute periods and the time taken in a series of eight trials on the Track Tracer.

In each case an estimate of the evenness of improvement is scored in terms of 'relapses'. A 'relapse' is defined as any trial which takes longer than a previous trial; the amount of the 'relapse' is the difference in output or time between two such adjacent trials. In the case of the test of concentration a 'relapse' occurs when less figures are produced than in a previous trial; the amount of the 'relapse' is the decrease in the number of figures.

In the measurement of tempo of tapping, where only four trials are given, the measure used is the variation of each of the four periods from the average of the four.

TESTS RELATED TO INTROVERSION

7. *The Tendency to exhibit Speed rather than Accuracy*

We have obtained evidence of the patient's preference, after leucotomy, for speed rather than accuracy, from a number of different approaches. We attempted to measure it specifically with regard to the performance on the Track Tracer. This machine has been described under (2). The patient is told that this is to test his skill and that he is to perform the task as *quickly* and as *accurately* as he can, both words being equally stressed. Eight trials are given on this machine.

In the analysis of the data, the first trial is ignored. Evidence of an increase in speed and the number of mistakes made comes from a comparison of these two variables before and after the operation. In addition the ratio of speed to accuracy is calculated.

We also found that the increase in speed and decrease in accuracy was noticeable on the non-verbal intelligence test we had used, the Porteus Mazes. This test was given in the prescribed manner, but the amount of time which was taken over each trial, on each of the ten mazes, was noted. A comparison of the total time taken to complete all the mazes was used in estimating the increased speed of the post-leucotomy patient.

Evidence of an increase in mistakes also came from the word-building test (17). In this test patients are asked to make as many words as they can out of a nine-letter word. Any word which they misspell or repeat, or which is non-existent, is counted as a mistake.

We also obtained evidence of an increase in speed in the rating of pictorial humour. In this test (10), which will be described in detail later, twenty-five pictorial jokes which had been collected from various picture papers have to be listed as either extremely amusing, amusing, slightly amusing or not amusing. The patient has to decide what he thinks about each joke, and then place it under one of the four cards on which are written the categories given above. A comparison of the speed with which he does this before and after the operation gives evidence of an increase in the speed of decision on this particular task.

8. *The Tendency towards Self-blame*

(a) *Intropunitive reactions to own incapacities*

The list of undesirable personality traits described under (4) was used to arrive at a measure of this tendency. If the patient considers himself to be characterised by any of these traits he is asked whether he blames himself for this characteristic. The total number of items for which he blames himself is calculated. In addition, the total number of unpleasant characteristics for which he does not blame himself is also calculated.

When the patient states that he blames himself for a particular characteristic, he is asked to try and estimate whether he blames himself *exceedingly, very much* or *a little*. We are thus able to estimate the intensity of the self-blame as subjectively reported by the patient.

A comparison of the number of items for which the patient blames himself before and after the operation is the measure of the change in the extent of self-blame; a comparison of the traits for which he blamed himself exceedingly, very much or a little produced the measure of the intensity of the blame.

(b) *Reaction to external frustration: an insoluble task*

After the patient has done ten mazes in the Porteus series, over each of which he could take as long as he liked, he is given an insoluble maze. He is told that he will have only 30 seconds to complete it, and that if he makes a mistake he should jump back to the centre. The path is traced with a stylus that does not mark the paper. The time limit is imposed to prevent the patient ascertaining that there is no solution to the maze. When the maze is taken away, the patient is told, 'You know that today I have been interested in what you think; I am not interested in what you have been told or what others think about you. Now please tell me why you think you could not do the last maze?' The patient's replies are noted down before and after the operation.

9. *Attitude to Time*

The subjective attitude to the past, present and future of patients before and after leucotomy is obtained from their answers to eight questions based on Israeli's (1936) work. These questions and answers are given verbally, the patient having the alternative answers past, present and future printed on a card in front of him.

1. Which do you think about most—the (*a*) past, (*b*) present or (*c*) future?
2. Which do you think about least?
3. Which do you feel least unhappy about?
4. Which do you feel most unhappy about?
5. Which do you worry about most?
6. Which do you worry about least?
7. Which are you most interested in?
8. Which are you least interested in?

A change in attitude is reported when it is shown by a significant percentage of the patients.

10. *Appreciation of Sex Humour*

(*a*) A number of pictorial jokes were collected from such magazines as the *New Yorker*, *Razzle*, *Men Only* and *Punch*. After some preliminary work, twenty-five of the jokes were selected, including both sex and neutral jokes, and were pasted on to pieces of cardboard. On each of four cards was printed in block capitals—'Extremely amusing', 'Amusing', 'Slightly amusing' and 'Not amusing' respectively; these four cards are placed next to each other in front of the patient, and the pile of jokes, in random order, is placed on his right-hand side.

The patient is asked to decide into which of these four categories he would place each of the jokes. He is to pick them up one at a time and place them face downwards below the card which he considers best describes it. The time taken to complete all twenty-five is noted on a stopwatch. The jokes are numbered and a note is made of the jokes appearing in each category for each of the patients.

The change following on leucotomy is ascertained by noting what had happened to each of the twenty-five jokes; that is, what percentage of the patients had changed their rating from category 'Not amusing' to 'Amusing' or 'Slightly amusing' to 'Not amusing' and so on.

A joke is classed as moving up the scale where the percentage of patients' rating moving up is significantly greater than the percentage moving down.

The jokes that were found to be moving up were then shown independently to three psychiatrists for a confirmation of their sexual content to correct for any bias in the investigator. The same confirmation was sought with regard to the jokes classed by the experimenter as neutral.

(b) The total number of jokes in each category was also compared before and after leucotomy.

11. *Endurance*

The test of physical endurance used is one which has been shown to be highly related to the factor of 'endurance' (Himmelweit and Petrie, 1951). It has also been shown to differentiate consistently between introverts and extraverts (Petrie, 1948A). For this test the patient is seated on a chair without a back-rest, and a second chair of the same height as the first is placed in front of and about 2 feet away from the patient. He is asked to place his outstretched right leg, with the knee straight, in such a position that the foot rests on the second chair. The other leg is resting on the floor and the hands are placed in the lap. In order to prevent the patient from seeking support from the wall or by leaning back, the chair on which the patient is seated is 2 inches from the wall behind him.

The patient is asked to raise his outstretched leg approximately 2 inches from the seat of the chair and to put it down again immediately. He is then asked to do this again, but this time to keep the leg in this position for as long as he can without leaning back. The time that he can successfully do this is measured on a stopwatch and constitutes his score on this test.

12. *Level of Aspiration*

(a) *Tendency to aim at a goal beyond their ability*

To arrive at a measure of the patient's goal-setting behaviour, the Track Tracer described under (3) is used. The patient is first given a practice trial. After the second trial he is asked to guess how long he has taken and how many mistakes he has made. When he has done this he is asked how long he thinks he will take next time, and how many mistakes he thinks he will make. A further trial is then completed. Again the patient is asked to estimate how long he has taken and how many mistakes he has made. After this he is told—for the first time—his actual score in time and mistakes.

Then he is asked to state how long he thinks he will take and how many mistakes he will make on the next trial. This procedure is repeated after each of the trials.

A measure of the goal-setting behaviour of the patient is obtained by comparing the achievement on the completed trial with the estimate of the future trial. This is done for each of the eight trials and the total of these is the goal discrepancy. The calculations are carried out separately with regard to time and mistakes. In addition, the 'blind' estimate made after the trial at which the real score was not divulged is compared with the 'blind' judgment.

An individual with a high level of aspiration sets his goal above his previous performance; that is, he thinks he will make fewer mistakes and do the task more quickly than he has achieved in the trial just completed.

(b) *Tendency to underrate performance when completed*

A comparison is made between the score achieved and the patient's estimate of this on each trial; the total of these for all trials is the judgment discrepancy. These scores are calculated separately for speed and mistakes. A patient who underestimates his performance tends to consider that he has made more mistakes and taken longer than has actually been the case. A separate calculation is made for the 'blind' judgment when the patient has as yet no knowledge of the actual time or mistakes.

13. *Fluctuation or Reversal of Perspective*

The Necker Cube is used for this test. This is a drawing of a cube without shading of any kind, which tends to be seen first from one angle and then from another. After the phenomenon has been explained to the patient, he is given a trial period in which he is asked to notice whether the cube shifts. When he understands what type of shift in the picture is experienced, he is asked to concentrate on the centre of the cube and to tap with his pencil after the cube shifts. He is not to try to cause it to shift, but just let it happen for the period of one minute which was measured on a time-interval clock The patient is then asked to try to make the cube shift as often as possible during a further period of one minute, and to tap with his pencil whenever the cube shifts.

We obtain the following scores from these tests: the number of 'unwilled' fluctuations in one minute, as measured during the first period; the number of 'willed' fluctuations as measured during the second minute; and the difference between the number of 'willed' and 'unwilled' fluctuations—the last score is used as a measure of his control in this situation.

14. *Concentration and Distractibility*

The patient is told he is going to be given a test of concentration. A series of figures will be read out and will be interrupted at irregular intervals by the word 'now'. When this occurs the patient is to try and repeat the last six numbers in the order in which they were read. The example is given that if the patient hears 5, 8, 3, 6, 4, 2, 1, 9, 5 'now', he should repeat 6, 4, 2, 1, 9 5, or as many of these six numbers as he can remember, in the right order. The instructions are modified and repeated if there is any doubt about the patient grasping what is required. Eight sets of numbers are read out, at the rate of two per second, and the patient's answers noted. The score is one point for each number remembered in the right sequence.

To obtain a measure of distractibility, the test of concentration is repeated to the accompaniment of a bell which sounds like a raucous telephone bell. A different series of numbers is used but the length of each series is the same. The score is the same as used in the test of concentration, the total score is the total number remembered.

The measure of distractibility is the difference between the scores with and without the distraction of the telephone bell.

The total number of figures repeated—irrespective of their correctness—was also calculated for the concentration and distractibility tests, and the number of mistakes was noted.

15. *Time Judgment*

(a) *Unfilled time*

The patient is told that a period of 15 seconds will be measured on a stopwatch. He will be given an indication of the beginning and end of the period by taps with a pencil on the table. He is to try to measure a further period of 15 seconds and tap with his pencil when he thinks it is over. He is asked not to count even in his head during the test. The explanation is modified and repeated until the patient fully understands what is required. The period which the patient regards as 15 seconds is noted.

The procedure is repeated for a period of one minute and again the patient's estimate is noted. The score used is the difference between the patient's estimation of a minute before and after the operation.

(b) *Filled time*

The second trial on the Track Tracer—which was described under 'Tests related to Neuroticism' (3)—is given without the patient being told of the actual time he has taken. He is asked to estimate how long this period has been (it varied between 30 seconds and 1½ minutes). The score used is the difference between the time he has actually taken and the time he thinks he has taken. A comparison is made between this difference before and after the operation.

16. *Fluency*

(a) The patient is asked to name as many round things as he can in a period of a minute. He is told, for example, that a penny is round and that anything round will do. The period is marked on a time-interval clock; the score is the number of items enumerated.

(*b*) The patient is presented with a drawing of a tree. He is asked to name as many different things as possible that could be found in such a picture in the position of an 'X' mark drawn under the tree. The procedure and score are identical with that in (*a*). Both tests are described by Cattell (1936).

17. *Persistence at a Task*

A card with the word EDUCATORS printed in block capitals is placed before the patient. The instructions given are as follows: 'You see this word? It has many letters in it. Each letter is different from the others. You will see that out of the three letters C A T one can make the word "cat". One can make different words out of these other letters. I want you to try to make as many words as you can and write them on your paper, one under the other, only using the letters in this word, but using as many of these letters or as few as you want. But you can't use any of the letters twice in the same word. Now make as many words as you can, and tell me when you are finished.' The time is noted when he has finished and the number of words is also noted; these are the two scores from this test.

18. *Attitude to Illness*

The patient is asked whether he thinks he is ill. His answer, with qualifications where present, is noted. It is explained to the patient that what is required is his real opinion, not the opinion of other people—however much he respects them. If his answer is positive he is asked whether he thinks he will get better. The number of patients who regard themselves as being ill, and the number who regard themselves as unlikely to get better, is compared before and after the operation.

ADDITIONAL TESTS USED FOR ROSTRAL PATIENTS

19. *Worries*

The Worry Questionnaire consists of a hundred items arranged in groups of five. The patient underlines anything about which he has been worried, nervous or anxious at this time of his life. The score is the number of items underlined.

20. *Interests*

The Interest Questionnaire consists of a hundred items which are arranged in twenty groups of five. Each of the items represents an interest which is found in some sections of the population. The patient is instructed to read through the list and underline everything he is interested in at that time of his life. He is to underline as many or as few items as he wishes and to do so at his own speed.

21. *Annoyances*

In the Annoyance Questionnaire there are twenty-eight items which might be found annoying. The patient is told that he is to underline any item which tends to annoy him at that time to his life. The score was the number of items underlined.

N.B. The Worry, Interest and Annoyance Questionnaires are adaptations of the Pressey X–O Test.

22. *Self-inventory based on Cattell's Factors of Neuroticism (C) and Introversion (F)*

Each patient was asked to answer a stencilled list of questions as follows:

Factor C
  1. Are you frequently in low spirits?
  2. Are you lonesome, even with others?
  3. Do you frequently feel grouchy?
  4. Do you get discouraged easily?
  5. Do you feel adjusted to life?

Factor F
  1. Are you often just miserable (for no reason)?
  2. Do you worry over possible misfortunes?
  3. Do you have frequent ups and downs of mood?
  4. Are you meditative and introspective?
  5. Are you carefree and can you relax?

A comparison was made of answers before and after the operation.

APPENDIX B

STATISTICAL TABLES

CHANGES THREE MONTHS AFTER BILATERAL POSTERIOR STANDARD LEUCOTOMY

(Twenty Patients)

	Mean difference	Standard deviation of difference	Critical ratio
TESTS RELATED TO NEUROTICISM			
Suggestibility			
(a) Suggestibility (sway with suggestion)	−2·35	4·04	2·33*
(b) Suggestibility (sway without suggestion)	−0·66	1·98	1·35
Suggestibility (a) − (b)	−1·69	3·66	1·84
Perseveration Ratio			
Reversed words	−1·88	4·18	1·90
Reversed figures (2, 3, 4)	0·09	2·59	N.S.
Manual Dexterity			
Highest score on Track Tracer (time)	−3·40	2·42	6·14*
Speed of Writing (number of letters per minute)	−3·70	14·18	N.S.
Self-criticism (number of undesirable traits)	−5·95	9·85	2·63*
Smoothness of Work Curves			
In tapping (variation from average)	−5·89	10·40	2·34*
On Track Tracer (amount of relapse)	−2·1	6·97	1·31
TESTS RELATED TO INTROVERSION			
Speed			
Mazes (total time)	−2·72	4·26	2·47*
Humour (speed of decision)	31·77	211·53	0·52
Wechsler Arithmetic (total time)	−55·50	74·21	3·08*
Wechsler Object Assembly (total time)	−10·38	79·90	0·50
Track Tracer (total time on all trials)	−45·75	51·52	3·87*
Track Tracer (time of second trial)	11·20	14·72	3·31*
Track Tracer (time of penultimate trial)	−8·55	13·24	2·81*

* Significant differences marked thus.   N.S. = Not significant.

CHANGES THREE MONTHS AFTER POSTERIOR LEUCOTOMY

	Mean difference	Standard deviation of difference	Critical ratio
Accuracy			
Mazes (number of failures)	1·82	2·38	3·25*
Wechsler Arithmetic (number of mistakes)	0·39	0·92	1·77
Track Tracer (number of mistakes on penultimate trial)	1·75	5·65	1·35
Persistence at a task (number of errors)	1·59	4·27	1·49
Speed/Accuracy Ratio			
Ratio of time to mistakes (trial 2)	−5·59	20·34	1·10
Ratio of time to mistakes (penultimate trial)	−3·95	22·86	0·67
Self-blame			
Total number of traits with blame	−4·58	7·66	2·53*
Blame exceedingly	−2·58	3·08	3·53*
Blame very much	−1·84	4·74	1·64
Blame a little	−0·16	5·42	0·12
Endurance			
Physical endurance (leg)	−20·89	30·50	2·82*
Attitude to Humour	Increased rating of sex jokes in comparison with neutral jokes*		
Attitude to Time	Increased interest and happiness in present (and future) as opposed to past*		
MISCELLANEOUS PERSONALITY TESTS			
Fluctuation (with effort)	6·47	11·54	2·24*
Fluctuation (without effort)	1·39	5·49	1·05
Concentration (number correct)	−0·74	10·23	0·31
Distractibility (number correct)	1·82	10·84	0·67
Concentration—Distractibility (number correct)	−1·94	11·38	0·66
Time estimation (60 seconds)	−1·50	20·88	0·29
Estimation of time taken on Track Tracer (1)	−15·0	70·75	0·92
Fluency (Round Articles)	−1·35	4·27	1·38
Fluency (Cattell Tree Picture)	−0·89	5·91	N.S.
Track Tracer (difference between second and penultimate speed)	2·50	14·65	0·74

* Significant differences marked thus.

CHANGES THREE MONTHS AFTER POSTERIOR LEUCOTOMY

	Mean difference	Standard deviation of difference	Critical ratio
INTELLECTUAL TESTS			
Wechsler Scale			
Verbal I.Q.	−7·21	6·35	4·81 *
Performance I.Q.	−0·34	6·10	0·24
Full-scale I.Q.	−4·82	5·10	4·02 *
Comprehension sub-test	−2·83	2·62	4·42 *
Digits sub-test	−0·32	2·65	0·52
Digits (numbers forward–backwards)	0·44	1·76	1·02
Arithmetic sub-test	−0·89	2·40	1·56
Similarities sub-test	−0·61	1·79	1·42
Object Assembly sub-test	−0·50	2·50	0·85
Digit Symbol sub-test	0·32	2·00	0·68
Picture Arrangement	−0·17	1·86	0·38
Picture Completion	−0·58	1·35	1·81
Porteus Mazes I.Q.	−12·79	17·25	3·14 *
Proverbs	Decrease in generalisation*		

* Significant differences marked thus.

CHANGES NINE MONTHS AFTER BILATERAL POSTERIOR STANDARD LEUCOTOMY

(*Twenty patients*)

	Mean difference	Standard deviation of difference	Critical ratio
TESTS RELATED TO NEUROTICISM			
Suggestibility			
(a) Suggestibility (sway with suggestion)	−2·91	3·99	2·91*
(b) Suggestibility (sway without suggestion)	−0·12	1·07	0·44
Suggestibility (a) − (b)	−2·79	3·89	2·88*
Perseveration ratio			
Reversed figures (2, 3, 4)	−0·72	1·46	2·12*
Manual Dexterity			
Highest score on Track Tracer (time)	−6·75	7·43	3·95*
Speed of Writing (number of letters per minute)	7·55	13·56	2·43*
Self-criticism (number of undesirable traits)	−6·84	10·12	2·86*
Smoothness of Work Curve			
In tapping (variation from average)	−1·39	14·93	0·39
On Track Tracer (amount of relapse)	0·05	16·83	0·03
TESTS RELATED TO INTROVERSION			
Speed			
Mazes (total time)	−1·14	3·42	1·30
Humour (speed of decision)	−57·13	139·74	1·53
Wechsler Arithmetic (total time)	−54·74	90·06	2·58*
Wechsler Object Assembly (total time)	−54·00	93·35	2·24*
Track Tracer (total time on all trials)	−54·45	45·82	5·18*
Track Tracer (time of second trial)	−16·70	15·09	4·83*
Track Tracer (time of penultimate trial)	−8·90	10·31	3·76*
Accuracy			
Mazes (number of failures)	0·70	2·15	1·43
Wechsler Arithmetic (number of mistakes)	0·68	1·00	2·83*
Track Tracer (total number of mistakes on all trials)	5·55	18·25	1·32
Track Tracer (total number of mistakes on penultimate trial)	1·75	4·60	1·67
Persistence at a task (number of errors)	3·94	13·20	1·19
Speed/Accuracy Ratio			
Ratio of time to mistakes (trial 2)	−8·89	22·16	1·75

* Significant differences marked thus.

CHANGES NINE MONTHS AFTER POSTERIOR LEUCOTOMY

	Mean difference	Standard deviation of difference	Critical ratio
Ratio of time to mistakes (penultimate trial)	−9·30	23·75	1·71
Self-blame			
Total number of traits with blame	−7·84	9·97	3·34*
Blame exceedingly	−1·89	4·19	1·91
Blame very much	−2·89	5·59	2·19*
Blame a little	−3·11	3·68	3·57*
Endurance			
Physical endurance (leg)	−13·94	23·09	2·42*
Attitude to Humour	Increased rating of sex jokes in comparison with neutral jokes*		
Attitude to Time	Increased interest and happiness in present (and future) as opposed to past*		
MISCELLANEOUS PERSONALITY TESTS			
Fluctuation (with effort)	5·06	10·33	1·90
Fluctuation (without effort)	−1·12	7·84	0·55
Fluctuation (with—without effort)	6·19	9·06	2·65*
Concentration (number correct)	1·95	7·90	1·05
Concentration (jaggedness of curve)	−2·80	9·01	1·16
Distractibility (number correct)	0·11	8·61	0·05
Distractibility (jaggedness of curve)	0	9·73	0
Concentration—Distractibility (number correct)	2·50	6·64	1·55
Time estimation (60 seconds)	1·18	22·95	0·22
Estimation of time taken on Track Tracer (1)	−6·80	41·54	0·71
Fluency (Round Articles)	0·20	5·43	0·16
Fluency (Cattell Tree Picture)	1·16	7·14	0·69
Track Tracer (difference between second and penultimate speed)	−3·45	8·75	1·72
INTELLECTUAL TESTS			
Wechsler Scale			
Verbal I.Q.	−7·51	10·31	3·09*
Performance I.Q.	1·49	6·05	1·04
Full-scale I.Q.	−3·57	6·77	2·23*
Comprehension sub-test	−2·17	2·83	3·14*

* Significant differences marked thus.

CHANGES THREE MONTHS AFTER POSTERIOR LEUCOTOMY

	Mean difference	Standard deviation of difference	Critical ratio
Comprehension Question:			
1 (Losing a book)	0·06	0·64	0·38
2 (Building a house)	−0·33	0·59	2·36*
3 (Preventing a train accident)	−0·39	0·61	2·60*
4 (Giving money to organised charity)	−0·61	0·61	4·07*
5 (Helping a good friend)	−0·06	0·64	0·38
6 (Treatment of criminals)	−0·44	0·86	2·10*
7 (Filling Government positions)	−0·22	0·43	2·20*
8 (Acquiring British citizenship)	−0·17	0·79	0·89
9 (Using cotton to make cloth)	0·17	0·86	0·81
10 (Keeping promises)	−0·56	0·78	2·95*
Digits sub-test	−0·16	3·82	0·18
Digits (numbers forwards–backwards)	0·37	2·41	0·65
Arithmetic sub-test	−1·26	2·81	1·91
Similarities sub-test	−0·72	1·99	1·50
Object Assembly sub-test	0	2·01	0
Digit Symbol sub-test	0·84	2·06	1·71
Picture Arrangement	−0·17	2·68	0·26
Picture Completion	−0·05	0·91	0·24
Porteus Mazes I.Q. (mental age)	−0·80	2·10	1·67
Proverbs	Decrease in generalisation*		

* Significant differences marked thus.

STATISTICAL TABLES
CHANGES SIX MONTHS AFTER BILATERAL ANTERIOR ROSTRAL LEUCOTOMY
(Fifteen patients)

	Mean difference	Standard deviation of difference	Critical ratio
TESTS RELATED TO NEUROTICISM			
Suggestibility			
(a) Suggestibility (sway with suggestion)	−2·65	4·21	2·27*
(b) Suggestibility (sway without suggestion)	0·27	0·66	1·47
Suggestibility (a) − (b)	−2·92	4·42	2·38*
Perseveration Ratio			
Reversed figures (2, 3, 4)	−0·72	1·35	1·85*
Manual Dexterity			
Highest score on Track Tracer (time)	−9·77	13·35	2·64*
Speed of Writing (number of letters per minute)	−13·43	10·75	4·67*
Self-criticism (number of undesirable traits)	−5·00	6·16	2·93*
TESTS RELATED TO INTROVERSION			
Speed			
Mazes (total time)	−9·37	23·45	1·44
Humour (speed of decision)	−128·23	182·93	2·53*
Wechsler Arithmetic (total time)	−71·14	105·37	2·53*
Track Tracer (total time on all trials)	−59·38	72·66	2·95*
Track Tracer (time of second trial)	−14·85	21·05	2·55*
Track Tracer (time of penultimate trial)	−10·38	13·34	2·81*
Accuracy			
Mazes (number of failures)	0·62	1·45	1·54
Wechsler Arithmetic (number of mistakes)	−0·50	1·40	1·34
Track Tracer (total number of mistakes on all trials)	4·92	27·38	0·65
Track Tracer (total number of mistakes on penultimate trial)	0·77	6·60	0·42
Persistence at a task (number of errors)	−0·29	4·76	0·23
Concentration (number of errors)	2·00	7·85	0·88
Speed/Accuracy Ratio			
Ratio of time to mistakes (trial 2)	−0·98	36·89	0·10
Ratio of time to mistakes (penultimate trial)	−1·35	18·14	0·27
Self-blame			
Total number of traits with blame	−2·33	3·89	2·07*

* Significant differences marked thus.

133

	Mean difference	Standard deviation of difference	Critical ratio
Blame exceedingly	−0·25	3·33	0·26
Blame very much	−1·33	4·46	1·03
Blame a little	−0·33	2·74	0·42
Endurance			
Physical endurance (leg)	3·43	13·75	0·93
Dynamometer grip	−0·78	15·03	0·16
Attitude to Humour	Increased rating of sex jokes in comparison with neutral jokes*		
Attitude to Time	Increased interest and happiness in present (and future) as opposed to past*		
MISCELLANEOUS PERSONALITY TESTS			
Fluctuation (with effort)	7·25	9·56	2·62*
Fluctuation (without effort)	1·92	8·31	0·80
Fluctuation (with—without effort)	5·33	7·13	2·59*
Concentration (number correct)	1·92	2·69	2·58*
Concentration (jaggedness of curve)	2·17	7·86	0·96
Distractibility (number correct)	1·85	6·01	1·11
Distractibility (jaggedness of curve)	2·42	4·44	1·89*
Concentration—Distractibility (number correct)	0·08	6·45	0·04
Time estimation (15 seconds)	4·35	6·97	1·97*
Time estimation (60 seconds)	10·33	10·15	3·05*
Estimation of time taken on Track Tracer (1)	−1·08	5·05	0·74
Fluency (Round Articles)	0·93	6·22	0·56
Fluency (Cattell Tree Picture)	1·15	3·41	1·22
Track Tracer (difference between second and penultimate speed)	−4·77	12·42	1·39
INTELLECTUAL TESTS			
Wechsler Scale			
Verbal I.Q.	2·02	6·75	1·12
Performance I.Q.	5·02	11·35	1·65
Full-scale I.Q.	3·09	9·56	1·21
Comprehension sub-test	−0·21	2·01	0·39
Comprehension Question:			
1 (Losing a book)	0·07	0·62	0·42
2 (Building a house)	0	0·68	0
3 (Preventing a train accident)	0·29	0·99	1·09

*Significant differences marked thus.

STATISTICAL TABLES

CHANGES SIX MONTHS AFTER ANTERIOR LEUCOTOMY

	Mean difference	Standard deviation of difference	Critical ratio
4 (Giving money to organised charity)	−0·07	0·73	0·36
5 (Helping a good friend)	0·21	0·58	1·36
6 (Treatment of criminals)	0	0·55	0
7 (Filling Government positions)	−0·07	0·62	0·42
8 (Acquiring British citizenship)	−0·14	0·53	0·98
9 (Using cotton to make cloth)	0·29	0·47	2·31*
10 (Keeping promises)	−0·36	0·63	2·13*
Digits sub-test	−0·14	2·03	0·26
Digits (number forwards—backwards)	0·29	1·94	0·56
Arithmetic sub-test	1·21	2·01	2·25*
Similarities sub-test	1·15	1·28	3·24*
Object Assembly sub-test	1·25	2·76	1·69
Digit Symbol sub-test	1·50	3·01	1·86*
Porteus Mazes I.Q.	1·15	12·51	0·33
Proverbs	No decrease in generalisation		

* Significant differences marked thus.

APPENDIX C   EXAMPLES OF PATIENTS' PRODUCTIONS

C.1. SAMPLES OF ANSWERS TO COMPREHENSION QUESTIONS BEFORE AND AFTER STANDARD LEUCOTOMY

	Before	After
What is the thing to do if you lose a book belonging to a library?		
Sophie	I'd go back and tell them I'd lost their book, and go to different places where I'd been.	Inform the stationmaster, let the police know and the Post Office where you have lost it from.
What is the thing to do if you lose a watch you have borrowed from a friend?		
Pauline	Tell her. I expect you would have to pay for the loss of it.	Borrow another watch.
What should you do if you see a train approaching a broken track?		
Felicity	Try and stop the train. Don't know how; tell a porter or someone connected with the railway.	Tell the nearest porter.
Gertrude	If a signal was not near, try and stop it yourself, waving your arms and so on.	You want to inform the person who could prevent the train from coming to it.
Josephine	Try and halt it in some way.	Stop it, but I don't know how. Go to a signalman, I suppose, but there might not be one there.
Horace	Try and flag it to a standstill.	Try and stop it. If unsuccessful, call the police.

136

James	Shout out if you can make the driver hear. Wave your arms—get on the track if not electric. Don't stay there too long.	Shout very loudly at the driver if I was in hearing distance of him.
Harry	If you have got something red hold it out and try and stop it, or stand on the track and try and stop it.	Stop it, I daresay.
Yolande	Try and get to a signal box, or if impossible wave something in front of the engine driver and stop train in time.	If I was in a position would try and warn them. If not, would try to get to the office and not to stand on the line.
George	Take off my coat or anything else, wave it, dash to the track to attract the attention of the driver.	Run down the line and attract the attention of the driver.
Pauline	Inform somebody in charge who could put the signal against. Give a signal to driver yourself if it was quicker.	Try to inform somebody who could do something about stopping the train.
Sophie	See if you could find a guard or porter, give some information or signal. Give an alarm.	Inform them at once. Trouble coming ahead if nothing is done. See the stationmaster.
Barbara	Theoretically, wave a red flag. Warn the driver by waving something red, or something you have on.	Wave a red flag in front of the train.
Rhoda	Warn the nearest person who is capable of helping or going to the nearest signal box.	Go to the nearest railway station and inform whoever is in charge. Stationmaster, I should think.

	Before	After
Why is it generally better to give money to an organised charity than to a street beggar?		
Kate	You are more certain it is going to a right cause, because the street beggar might be making money and playing on your sympathy.	You know where the money goes.
Cynthia	An authorised organisation is really doing good, but a beggar might not be putting it to the purpose you think he is.	To give to a street beggar though they may need it, they haven't got a licence. Door-to-door beggars must have a licence.
What should you do if a very good friend asks you for something you have not got?		
Doris	Try and obtain it from somewhere for them.	Tell the person to ask a friend that you know would be able to help them.
Selina	Try and get it for them.	Tell them I hadn't got it, and therefore couldn't lend it.
Janet	Try and get it for her.	Say you haven't got it.
Pauline	Try and get it for them. Say you are sorry you can't give it to them.	Tell them you haven't got it.
Sophie	Have to let her down. If you haven't got it you can't give it. Do the second best, give her something like what she was asking for.	If you haven't got it, you haven't got it.
Rhoda	If it was very necessary I would try and procure it.	Tell them you haven't got it.

138

Why are criminals locked up or put in prison?

Kate	Because they are a menace to the public, and because they must undergo some form of punishment.	Because they are a nuisance to others.
Felicity	In case they should repeat the offence, and also for punishment.	Because they have done something wrong.
Gertrude	To prevent further misdeeds and punish them for what they have done wrong.	To punish them for what they have done wrong.
Josephine	Because of the safety of the public, and for their own punishment.	To save the rest of humanity. If you don't stop them they're liable to do it to everyone.
Horace	They're safe whilst in prison. Secondly, later on perhaps they will be different.	So that they can't do any more harm, I suppose.
James	First as a punishment, and as a deterrent to others.	It shows other people that if they commit crimes they are punished for them.
Pauline	Benefit of the public. Teach them a lesson not to do the same wrong again. To teach others not to do the same.	So that they shan't do further harm.
Claire	They're a danger to community. Help them to occupy their lives in a better way. Partly treatment.	So that they're not a public menace.
Rhoda	So that they can't damage anyone else or repeat their crime for a certain amount of time, apart from punishing them.	To prevent them doing more damage.

139

	Before	After
Why should Government posts be filled through Civil Service examinations?		
Kate	Because it is necessary to see a person's capabilities and see whether they can fit into the job, and because a Government position is a responsible one.	Because the people can be sure that you are doing the job in the correct way.
Gertrude	So that they set a standard of training. People who go into the Civil Service should be up to a certain standard.	I don't know how to word it. It's silly to say they are all of the same education, because that isn't correct.
Why does the British Government make a person wait from the time he makes application until he receives his British citizenship?		
Doris	To make sure that the person is genuine.	I don't know.
George	From the period they apply they are under very severe scrutiny, and their past records are looked into and references taken up.	To look into a man's past history.
Pauline	Likelihood of person wanting to alter for the wrong reason. You have to check up on their life and nationality.	Takes a certain amount of time to organise these things.
Why should a promise be kept?		
Simon	Because there are fundamental laws of right and truth which each person is bound to obey; because any stable order in society depends on unwritten bonds as well as the written ones. It is bound up with the individual's self-respect.	Because keeping promises is an essential condition of stable life in a civilised community and leads to the recognition of the importance of truth and loyalty.

Felicity	It makes the person you promised it to unhappy and lose faith in you.	Just because it's a promise.
Doris	Because it would disappoint someone if you did not.	I can't think of that.
Horace	On principle. Once anybody does not, you don't trust them again.	In good faith—so that—on principle.
James	If one does not keep a promise it lowers one's own self-respect, and other people lose confidence in you.	Helps one's own self-respect if one keeps a promise.
Harry	You have a trust in a person and when you promise it says that you want to be trusted. It is a kind of a vow.	Usually vouch a promise and therefore it should be kept.
George	As a matter of honour. It is due to yourself firstly and secondly you cannot let down the other person.	A promise should always be kept.
Laura	It should be kept because one gives one's word for it.	Because it's something quite serious.
Barbara	In order not to disappoint other people.	To fulfil the hopes of other people.
Rhoda	If you have any sense of decency, it is usual to keep it if you have given your word of honour.	That is the object of making a promise, that you are going to keep it.

141

C.2. EXAMPLES OF TWO PATIENTS' ESSAYS BEFORE AND AFTER STANDARD LEUCOTOMY

Describe as accurately as you can a person (man or woman) you like very much; not his face or appearance, but what he is really like. Give initials and not a name. Take as long as you like.

Patient James before the Operation

'A man I like very much is a man whose initials are A. B. C. I knew him slightly before the war and have come in contact with him quite a lot since. He is married and has two small children, a boy aged three years and a girl now ten months old. He works for an insurance company and is about two years older than myself. He plays football in the Winter for a school Old Boy's club, and tennis in the Summer. He is a keen gardener.

'He is very interested in politics and business generally and we have had some long and interesting discussions on these matters.'

Patient James after the Operation

'Of the different people with whom I have come in contact from time to time I think the person—outside my own family—that I liked most was a man with whom I first became friendly when we were boys together at school. I can refer to him as A. B. C. although these are not his real initials.

'I can well remember my first conversation with him. We were both new boys that Summer Term and we happened to be standing next to each other in a queue of boys who were lining up to put their names down for new School blazers. It was one day during the first week of the term. We were rather restrained in our reactions, not nervous or apprehensive but subdued. We were thus pleased to find, after a few minutes' talk, that we were both in the same position. His dry but cheerful humour appealed to me, as also did the fact that he never made any attempt to impress people with any imagined super-qualities of his own.

'I think he rather lacked confidence as far as the academic side of school work was concerned, but he was a calm, agile and skilful games player. As I was always intensely keen on

142

running, tennis and cricket our mutual interest in these spheres formed an additional bond between us.

'A. B. C. left school about a term before I did. He became an articled clerk in his Uncle's solicitor's firm in Holborn. I kept up a continuous friendship with him in post-school years and often had lunch with him in town and went to shows together. We also enjoyed quite a number of games of golf at weekends. About 3 or 4 years after he left school A. B. C. joined the Territorial Unit and about a year later persuaded me to join the same regiment. Thereafter I naturally saw quite a lot of him, at H.Q. and the annual camp. I found that he showed then the qualities which had appealed to me from the first, namely a keen but cheerful sense of humour, modesty about his affairs and personal qualities, and vigorous interest in open-air pursuits. This latter characteristic led to rather a paradoxical situation for him, for having passed his Solicitor's Final examination about a year before the war, he then went out to Palestine where he joined the Palestine Police.'

Describe as accurately as you can a person (male or female) you dislike quite a lot; not his face or appearance, but what he is really like. Give initials and not a name. Take as long as you like.

Patient James before the Operation

'A man I dislike quite a lot is X. Y. Z. I knew him in the factory where I worked but have not come across him since I left that firm last year.

'He was the charge-hand of one of the benches whose work the Test department (for which I worked) had to inspect and was often inclined to be difficult about getting defects put right. My dislike of him arose from the fact that when pressed by those in authority over him he often became dishonest about what had been suggested. One came to the conclusion that he put his own position before the work he was handling.'

Patient James after the Operation

'I should say right away that in the ordinary course of events I am not given to taking a strong dislike to people. If I find a particular person's manner jars on me, my normal reaction is to avoid contact with that person as far as possible.

'There are some circumstances, of course, in which such "evading action" is not possible and this situation arose for a short time during the war when I was on the Test and Inspection department of a firm of electrical manufacturers. No foreman likes having his work rejected, but most foremen in that firm were fairly reasonable about having defective work put right. There was one man, however, whom I will call X. Y. Z., whose name was a by-word in the Test department for his obstinate refusal to co-operate.

'X. Y. Z. was very successful in bullying the men under him to work hard, but he would insist on adopting the same technique with the inspection assistants. The reason I disliked him was that he always took it as a personal affront when any of the work from his benches was rejected. Any such occurrence was made the occasion for personal abuse and the attempt to begin a violent harangue. As the inspection department was extremely busy at the time this added very much to the strain of the work. All this was particularly annoying as he knew perfectly well that before work finally left the factory it was subjected to a pretty thorough final check by the Government's own inspectors.'

Describe yourself as you think you would be seen by the person you described whom you like very much. Not your face or appearance, but what you are really like.

Patient James before the Operation

'I think A. B. C. looks on my activities with a certain good-natured tolerance. He lives a few doors down my road and we served at the same A.R.P. depot for several months. He proved a lot superior to me at tennis but I was able to have my revenge at table-tennis.

'Presumably he regards me, generally speaking, as of rather an unsociable turn of mind, in view of the fact that I invariably avoid dances, parties and other sociable gatherings.

'But I should think that he would credit me with a certain seriousness of mind and outlook about national and international affairs.'

Patient James after the Operation

'I have already described how A. B. C. and I first became

friendly (Ex. 1). As I have said he was a boy who suffered from a lack of confidence as far as his school work was concerned. As I myself was very slow in getting going in the sphere of school study we were both at about the same level in this respect. Later I passed him in work and reached the top positions in the form. He probably envied me in this respect. I expect he came to look upon me as having a more studious and perhaps more facile mind than himself, but since he had no academic ambitions there was nothing in this to affect our friendship. In any case at the same time he himself showed a slight but definite superiority to myself in games. Despite his success in sports A. B. C. formed few friendships—that with myself being the closest.

'Even after he left school he did not seem to make friends easily or quickly and was thus glad to maintain our association. This was in spite of the fact that he eventually had far more money to spend than myself, having come into a useful private income at the age of 21.

'I think A. B. C. looked upon me as being rather flippant in my attitude to life in general (though studious at work) and not as serious-minded as himself. But I believe he appreciated a sense of humour.'

Describe yourself as you think you would be seen by the person you described whom you dislike quite a lot; not your face or appearance but what you are really *like.*

Patient James before the Operation

'X. Y. Z. probably regarded me as almost a shade too conscientious about approving work submitted for Test and Inspection. He had a hearty detestation of the "theoretical" as opposed to the "practical" attitude to electrical manufacturing, and no doubt included my own leaning towards book work in that dislike. He represented one of the old practical die-hards who learn nothing by reading and everything by experience.'

Patient James after the Operation

'I do not think X. Y. Z. ever disliked me as much as I disliked him, since he treated all members of the Test bench in the same way.

'I am sure he looked upon me as officious, perhaps even over-conscientious. He undoubtedly considered me as obstinate in refusing to accept work which did not seem up to the required standard. Although he affected a contempt for the academic side of electrical engineering, in reality I believe he had a genuine respect for it, and I myself suffered through this as I was not attending evening classes at that time as some of my colleagues were doing. I think the thing he disliked most about me was my refusal to react to personal rudeness. I merely regarded that as part of the give and take of factory life, and consequently his efforts in that direction never made any impression on me.'

Describe as accurately as you can a person (man or woman) you like very much; not his face or appearance, but what he is really like. Give initials and not a name. Take as long as you like.

Patient Emily before the Operation

'Happy in the service of worthy men and women with whom she comes into contact. Denying herself. Hopeful of the future. Devoted to her family. Hardworking still although 80 years have passed since she first drew breath. A sunny nature. Patient in trials. Always making friends welcome, and those who come, and have come to her for help or advice. Loving her garden and flowers and home. Her initials are D. E. F.

'But how do I really write this? I know it is true, but somehow I do not seem able to prove my affection.'

Patient Emily after the Operation

'D. E. F. is a darling. She has known me all my life, and has always worked hard. She is generally the first one up in the morning, and last one to bed. Her health has always been good, and nothing seems too hard for her to attempt it. She is nearly 83 and is always ready to help anyone she knows. She is fond of gardening, and often is busy there until it is dark. Will she rest in the afternoon? No. There is always some little job to do. In fact we say we shall have to give her a duster when she dies. She is always busy here, and I suppose she will always want to feel she is ready for any emergency.'

EXAMPLES OF PATIENTS' PRODUCTIONS

*Describe as accurately as you can a person (man or woman) you dis-
like quite a lot; not his face or appearance, but what he is really like.
Give initials, not a name. Take as long as you like.*

Patient Emily before the Operation

'U. V. W. is a man I dislike quite a lot. He is married and his
wife and I were childhood friends. When visiting them once for
several days' stay, he forced me to sit on his knee and tried to
kiss me. During the past war in which he served in the A.R.P.
he was sometimes unable to travel to his home, some miles
away, and was given hospitality for the night by my parents.
The disliked actions were several times attempted during this
hospitality, and having taken a cup of tea to all at home before
their rising in the morning, as was my custom, I was asked on
more than one occasion by this man to have little clothing on.
Such behaviour by a man who had always appeared an admirable
character in every other way—and I had no reason to believe he
had any other bad points—has given me a strong dislike for him.'

Patient Emily after the Operation

'U. V. W. is a person whom I dislike. I knew him when we
were children. He subsequently became engaged to a friend of
mine, and was married to her. I was bridesmaid, and after some
time I was godmother to their child. She is entering the nursing
profession next January. U. V. W. was not serving in the
general forces during the recent war, but was engaged in Home
Guard duties and sometimes was too late to catch the last train
home. He would 'phone then and ask if he could come to stay
the night. He always could, of course, and would ask me to
bring in a cup of tea in the morning. After a few times he would
say—don't bother to dress first, and he seemed to like me to stay
chatting—but I did not wish to stay, as I had to be up and
doing, and help prepare his breakfast. And during the evening
he would try to get me to sit on his knee and to kiss me. I won't
even allow my own doctor to call me "dear" so I was not at all
pleased with the attentions of U. V. W.'

*Describe yourself as you think you would be seen by the person you
described whom you like very much, not your face or appearance, but
what you are really like. Take as long as you like.*

EXAMPLES OF PATIENTS' PRODUCTIONS

Patient Emily before the Operation

'I think I would be seen by the person I have described whom I like very much as very patient and punctual—a sincere friend—willing and anxious to do my very best at my work, and taking a great interest in my home, and longing to be there again. She must think me strangely unkind not to go to see her now.'

Patient Emily after the Operation

'Well, that depends on what I am doing. If I am playing the piano then I am the "Joy of Mother's heart". But if I am out doing someone else's shopping, and am a long time away, then it is suggested that I like Mrs. —— better than my mother. On the whole, however, I suppose I am considered "not a bad sort". She is pleased I am at home now, and can always find something for me to do for her.'

Describe yourself as you think you would be seen by the person you described whom you dislike quite a lot; not your face or your appearance, but what you are really like. Take as long as you like.

Patient Emily before the Operation

'I think I would be described by the person whom I disliked as he had previously known me—sincere to all my friends and honourable in every way. I think he would avoid describing my personality regarding my resistance to his despicable actions.'

Patient Emily after the Operation

'Goodness knows! I do not like U. V. W., but he has never shown dislike for me. There are many other people he could have contacted, but I suppose he thought he would be well received in my home, so I think he must have a good opinion of me.'

EXAMPLES OF PATIENTS' PRODUCTIONS

C.3. EXAMPLES OF PECULIARITIES OF LANGUAGE AND THOUGHT FOLLOWING ON STANDARD LEUCOTOMY

This material is derived from answers to the following sets of questions from the Wechsler Scale:

(a) *Comprehension questions*

1. What is the thing to do if you lose a book belonging to a library?
2. Why is it better to build a house with brick than wood?
3. What should you do if you see a train approaching a broken track?
4. Why is it generally better to give money to an organised charity than to a street beggar?
5. What is the thing to do if a very good friend asks you for something you don't have?
6. Why are criminals locked up or put in prison?
7. Why should most Government positions be filled through Civil Service examinations?
8. Why does Great Britain make a person wait from the time he makes application until the time he receives his citizenship?
9. Why is cotton used in making cloth?
10. Why should a promise be kept?

(b) *Similarities*

'I am going to name two things which are the same or alike in certain ways and I want you to tell me in what way they are alike. For example: In what way are a *plum* and a *peach* the same or alike?' (12 pairs of items.)

(c) *Vocabulary test*

'I want to see how many words you know. Listen carefully. When I say a word you tell me what it means. For example: What does *hero* mean?' (45 words.)

Note.—The answers before Standard leucotomy are presented side by side with the answers three months and nine months after the operation. Although some of these may be considered acceptable or even a vivid form of expression, it is hoped that this method of presentation will be helpful in evaluating the change that has taken place. Wechsler Verbal I.Q. is given in each case.

149

Question	Before leucotomy	Three months after Standard leucotomy	Nine months after Standard leucotomy
Simon *I.Q. 143* Hero	Man of outstanding courage who arouses in others respect and the desire to emulate.	A man of great attractive courage.	
Kate *I.Q. 99* Cat and mouse are alike because—	Keep up at night looking for food. Both on alert at night. Quick.	Seekers—usually for their food.	
Liberty—justice	Tends to free anybody. Common to law; desired.	Both states to be in when you're given permission to do as you please or restricted by time. Justice would be allowed to work or play as normal people.	
Box	Kind of case which you put things into. Four-sided figure—lid usually.	Usually four-sided figure in which you keep certain *quantities.*	
Umbrella	A protection which you use for rain.	A *utensil* used for when we have rainy weather to *shade* yourself.	
Belfry	Where they have bells, usually in towers, place where they keep them.	Usually used as a clock.	

150

Doris I.Q. 115 Question 2 Brave	House is made of brick because it lasts longer. Not afraid.	Lasts longer.	It is better for endurance. Unfrightened.
Gertrude I.Q. 113·5 Belfry	A balcony.		Belfry is your head; it must be because they say 'bats in the belfry'.
Josephine I.Q. 108 Question 8	They have to go into their case; there is so much red tape that I wonder they don't have to wait longer.		I suppose they have to *gee-up* that everything they have said is correct. I suppose you cannot go in one day and expect to be something the next day.
Diamond Cushion Umbrella Sword	Jewel. Article of comfort—pad. Article for keeping you dry. Used to kill with.	Just a pad. Covering. Instrument of torture.	Worthy jewel. Pad of comfort. Source of covering. An implement.
Horace I.Q. 110 Question 7	It would not be right for political leaders to choose people politically inclined to their way of thinking, anybody prejudiced or just one-sided.		It makes people unpolitical; gets people who are not political.

151

Question	Before leucotomy	Three months after Standard leucotomy	Nine months after Standard leucotomy
James I.Q. *129* Letter	Part of the alphabet or something you write to a friend.	An independent unit of the alphabet.	Something you send to friends or acquaintances which is really a collection of words.
Beatrice I.Q. *103* Bad	Something not pleasant. Unclean. Rotten.		Not too good.
Brave	To be able to face something which one dreads without hesitation—bold.		To show good taste.
Nuisance	Generally unpleasant.		To be a bit of a bother and a humbug—one as well as the other.
Fur	Pelt of an animal.		The coat on an animal which can be used as a wearing *apparatus.*
Nitroglycerine	Used for explosives.		Used for inventing—I think an explosive, you have got to find out these things.
Belfry	Where the bells of a church are kept.		An alcove where a bell lies.
Affliction	To be stricken with something.		To be *accosted* with something like an illness or something wrong with the body—just one eye or two.

			Something which might enter a balloon or room or anything.
Ballast	Used for weighing and lightening load of a balloon or aeroplane.		
Henry I.Q. 115 Ballast Question 9	Used in concrete—substance of sand and rubble. For thin cloth it is the only thing that could be used beside silk. It is pliable.	Some weight anywhere, cause of ballast. To keep it together and make a small job of it.	
Selina I.Q. 99·5 Question 4	Organised charity is the right thing to give it to and the street beggar you are not sure of.	You know it will go direct to the firm. It all means the same thing—go direct to the Company he was begging for.	
Janet I.Q. 115 Question 1	I would have to report it and they make a charge.	Report it to the library. I should have to advertise but could not get one back by doing that.	
Scissors—copper pan	They are both made of metal.	They are useful. Never seen a pair of scissors anything but scissors colour. Both made of metal of some kind.	

153

Question	Before leucotomy	Three months after Standard leucotomy	Nine months after Standard leucotomy
George I.Q. *130* Question 1	Report it at the library or be willing to pay for it after having made sure you cannot find it.		You should declare it.
Belfry	Upper part of a church housing bells.		Mechanical device used in defence or attack.
Seclude	To keep from.	To exclude.	To preclude.
Cynthia I.Q. *109·5* Question 4	An authorised organisation is really doing good, but a beggar might not be putting it to the purpose you thought he would.	It is recognised by people who run it, whereas organised beggar might not be as honest as you hope.	To give it to a street beggar, though they may need it they haven't got a licence. For door-to-door you must have a licence.
Question 7	Because they are fairly highly educated people; so that you get the best brains of the country to govern it.		People who qualify should be bright and know qualifications of people whom they are going to rule.
Hero	Someone who has done great deeds, achieved great things.	A man who has committed skill.	
Spangle	Article of jewellery which sparkles.	Shines or *flusters* or sparkles. Imitation jewellery.	
Affliction	To be maimed.	An aside. Affectation—people pretending what they are not.	

154

Sophie *I.Q. 100* Question 1	I'd go back and tell them I'd lost their book and go to different places where I'd been.	I would inform the *station-master*—let the police know and the Post Office where I'd lost it from.	
Roberta *I.Q. 118* Bad	Reverse of good—evil.	Something reversed good.	
Barbara *I.Q. 116* Question 2	There is less danger of fire, there is better insulation, less shrinkage and warping, etc		Bricks don't burn down as well as wood—keeps out extremes of temperature better than wood.
First—last Diamond	Limits to something. A form of carbon. It is a transparent precious stone.		Ends of performance. Carbon compounds used in *engineering capacities*. Transparent. Causing *reflection* of light. Normally cut with facets. Very hard.
Cushion	Soft. Two pieces of cloth stuffed with kapok or feathers for resting against.		Normally two squares of material joined at edges filled with soft material, down or Dunlop pillow or feathers to give comfort to *sitting* or *lying* *humans.*

155

Question	Before leucotomy	Three months after Standard leucotomy	Nine months after Standard leucotomy
Barbara *I.Q. 116* Belfry	Generally a tower where the bells are fixed.		Tower containing bells *from which bell-ringing comes.*
Ballast	A weight.		Weight carried by a ship or other *container.*
Nail	Flattened protective end to finger.		Metal joiner.
Flout	To deliberately disobey.		Set against the raising of some thing.
Richard *I.Q. 120* Fable	Legend.	A *far-reaching* tale, usually with moral attached. (Explained—going far back into history.)	
Dilatory	Slipshod.	Ship-shop.	
Sword	Fighting implement.		Metallic object. Metal flattened object which can be utilised for offensive purposes.

156

APPENDIX D

SAMPLES OF CASE HISTORIES

SAMPLE CASE HISTORIES OF FOUR LEUCOTOMY PATIENTS INCLUDED IN THE INVESTIGATIONS REPORTED IN THE PREVIOUS CHAPTER. These people were subjected to the following operations:

      (a) Standard
      (b) Standard
      (c) Bilateral Rostral
      (d) Unilateral Rostral

(a) Barbara, aged 37, was petite, and, when we first saw her, wore a sullen, pouting expression, and was obviously exceedingly worried and troubled. One had the impression that she would be very attractive when life was going more smoothly for her, although she now looked older than her age.

Barbara came of a middle-class family; her father was a senior civil servant. She had gone to a good school from where she obtained a scholarship to one of the leading universities and there obtained a first-class degree in biology. Barbara was sufficiently well thought of to be appointed to a teaching post in a public school. After a few years of teaching she married a man who had been divorced but who had retained the son of his first marriage. She had two children of her own, aged 4 and 9, when she came into hospital.

She is reported to have led a full social life at school and at the university, and she had many admirers. Her husband describes her as having been pleasant, sensible, intelligent and with plenty of friends. The testimonials from her university teachers and the headmistress of the school at which she taught were excellent and referred to her quick and orderly mind, her particular gifts as a teacher, her poise and her personality. They were convinced that she would go far; they found her equally pleasant as colleague or pupil.

On coming to see us she complained of serious headaches, difficulty both in getting off to sleep and staying asleep, and feeling abnormally tired and exhausted during the day. These symptoms had first started six years previously; now they were much more severe and she described herself as 'trembling all over'. She had been vomiting and when this ceased she continued to retch. She did not want to eat, and in her own words was 'in the depths of anguish'. She certainly had suicidal ideas, and kept a box of sleeping tablets by her side for this purpose. Any effort led to an increase of all these symptoms until finally she just stayed in bed for weeks on end.

As she did not respond to any other type of treatment when she came into hospital, it was decided to perform a Standard prefrontal leucotomy. This was done without complications. Some change in personality and improvement of symptoms were noted almost immediately after the operation. One month after, she was cheerful, co-operative and uninhibited, and was able to take part in ward social activities, including a play that was produced by the patients at Christmas time. Previously she had completely withdrawn herself from the life of the ward. Six weeks after the operation she stated 'that she was ready for anything'.

After three successful week-ends with her family she went home for good. Her energy was maintained and she was no longer troubled with incapacitating headaches and sleeplessness. Both the patient and her husband were delighted with the success of the operation.

Four months after the operation the husband, after a very successful holiday abroad, wrote, 'I should like to report on the condition of Barbara, and her sustained recovery. She enjoyed every minute of our holiday, fed like a horse, enjoyed flying and has come back determined to have chimneys swept, make new curtains, really look after the children and sooner or later go back to teaching.' A month later he wrote, 'Barbara is undoubtedly a much pleasanter companion to live with. Emotional rows are a thing of the past.'

When she came to see us there was also a remarkable change noticeable in her appearance. She obviously had taken great pains to make the best of herself and looked really pretty. There were many indications that she was interested in what was happening round her. She reported that she was sleeping better and appeared exceedingly grateful for all that had been done for her. There was also a marked difference in her co-operativeness in psychological examination in comparison with her pre-operative behaviour.

Relations with the stepson are reported by the husband to be more natural and friendly, and, indeed, affectionate. He also states that her sense of humour is restored.

The patient succeeded in obtaining a teaching post in a technical college, which she combined with looking after the home. She was responsible for the teaching of biology throughout the school, including a group of students working for the Oxford Senior Certificate. (Biology had not previously been taught at this school.) She also acted as form mistress to one of the senior forms. Barbara stated that she 'enjoyed teaching immensely'.

She remained at the technical college for one term (September to December). The reason she gave for resigning from this post was that full-time teaching and the strain of the long journey from home to school were too much for her. She hoped to find another appointment nearer home. In the testimonial which the headmistress provided at the end of the term, it was mentioned that Barbara had carried out all her duties conscientiously, that her discipline was good and that she taught thoroughly and effectively.

Eighteen months after the operation she came to the hospital for a demonstration to the medical staff, when she gave a coherent and optimistic account of her continued progress. She looked well cared for, happy and extremely presentable.

The patient's own spontaneous written description, entitled 'Changes in me due to Leucotomy', written fourteen months after the operation was as follows:

1. Much more physical strength and mental stamina than in the year before the operation.
2. Less emotional, but I think I am still more emotional than my husband.
3. I have lost what my husband calls my 'pathological unselfishness'.
4. Less tactful than I used to be—but this cannot be acute, as I was obviously well liked by most of the staff and girls at the school.

5. Extravagant. I thought that this came from the loss of unselfishness, but I realise now it is thoughtless spending.
6. I now miss my husband acutely when he is frequently away from London on his job. It was to counteract this that made me want to teach again.
7. Not now over-sensitive to other people's worries and troubles—now a lot harder.

(b) Simon, aged 30, was a cheerful, pleasant, rather shy young curate. He came of a middle-class family; his father was a retired civil servant. There were a number of other children, all healthy and contented. He went to an elementary school and then to a secondary school, and later obtained a first-class honours degree at a good university and entered a theological college. He had few friends at the university but acquired many at the theological college. After his training he was ordained and went to his first parish, where he was working when he came to see us. He lived in lodgings and was looked after by his landlady.

On coming to hospital Simon complained of symptoms which had developed insidiously ten years previously, had become more severe during the last two years and extremely troublesome during the last six months. He found it increasingly difficult to make decisions: for example, it would take him nearly an hour to decide whether or not he would go to the service which his vicar was taking the following morning. Eventually he found himself spending most of his day making up his mind how he ought to be spending his time, and by the time he had made up his mind the day was over. An increased amount of time was also spent in performing routine tasks; half an hour would be spent in setting the alarm clock. It was necessary for him repeatedly to wash his hands; whenever he touched anything he felt compelled to wash them all over again. He said that he was being troubled by unpleasant thoughts during his prayers, and at other times, and finally during the period when he was preaching. During his stay in hospital it was also noted that he spent the major part of the day in private prayer. He had to spend longer and longer over these daily prayers.

After a period of observation it was decided that there was no prospect of his returning to work without an operation. A Standard prefrontal leucotomy was performed. A change was perceptible almost immediately. The patient stated on the first day after the operation ' the strain has gone'.

Two months after the operation he preached a sermon without notes in the hospital chapel which was so effective that he was asked to give a sermon at the local church. He continued to preach at the hospital chapel until his discharge. He also arranged one evening's very successful entertainment at the hospital.

Four months after the operation we received a report from the friend with whom he was staying (himself a vicar) which said that the patient was extremely well in himself, that he had preached once or twice and done it well and had also taken services. At this period the patient stated to a friend that he was feeling very well—never better. This friend then suggested that, subject to our agreeing, Simon might again take on responsibility for a parish, and this he is now doing.

One year and nine months after leucotomy Simon came to see me. He stated that he thought he was much better than he had been nine months previously. He mentioned that he got 'a kick out of most things'. He enjoyed visiting, travelling and preaching. He thought he preached much better than he had done previously, and that he was more effective. He summed up by saying that he felt he had all the advantages and none of the disadvantages of the treatment.

The friend reports that he is happy in the parish, likes the work and is able to cope adequately with his duties.

(c) Ada, aged 42, was a clerk who had been with the same firm for more than twenty years. This is a small draper's establishment in a small town near London. At the time of the commencement of her illness the patient had been second in command of the clerical department. She is unmarried.

Ada's mother died at her birth, and she was brought up by a foster mother; her three siblings were looked after elsewhere. The foster mother had five children of her own, but was a real mother to Ada, who was extremely devoted to her until her death when Ada was 21. The foster father died eleven years later. For ten of these he had suffered from a nervous disorder in which he had been excited and obscene and paced about the house. The two foster sisters unmarried after the mother's death lived with Ada. One of these had been psychotic and had been living as a voluntary patient in a hospital part of the time. Ada suffered a great deal from the jealousy and spitefulness of this foster sister. The other foster sister has been Ada's best lifelong friend and continues to be attached to her.

Childhood in both home and school had been happy. Ada has always been a precise, over-conscientious, dogged, detail-loving person, easily worried by interference with her own routine, but friendly, cheerful and with no gross neurotic symptoms. The patient never had any sexual worries, interests or relationships. She stated that she was 'too occupied with the practical side of life' for this.

After the foster mother's death, and the foster father's mental illness, Ada lost interest in food; menstruation also ceased. There was also a restriction in interest in affairs outside of the house, but she remained at work and there is no indication that her efficiency decreased. At the age of 37, after an attack of influenza, she became depressed and feared she would be unable to do her work, so she stayed at home, a semi-invalid, for nearly two years. She then returned to work and remained there for eighteen months, after which she caught a cold, stayed away and did not return. Loss of weight and weakness increased; Ada then became an in-patient in hospital for four months, and she started to have pains in her stomach. The following year she was at home, whilst one foster sister was in and out of mental hospitals; the patient was always better when this foster sister was away.

Ada again went into hospital for six months, where she had E.C.T. and modified insulin treatment. On coming out her abdominal pains were worse and her appetite had dropped to almost nothing. Her sense of 'bottled up' agitation increased. When she was admitted to St. George's she complained that 'the nerves of the whole system were all agog' and of her loss of appetite. She explained that the cause of her illness was 'worry, due to rowing with my foster sister, who had always gone out of her way to be nasty because of her jealousy of the other foster sister's friendship for me.'

She was regarded as being in a state of advanced emaciation, resulting from anorexia nervosa over a period of twenty years, with considerable increase during the last year. As further deterioration in her condition might have proved fatal and there was no indication that she would respond to any other form of treatment, leucotomy was recommended. A prefrontal bilateral Rostral operation was carried out by Mr. McKissock. After the operation she slowly started to gain weight. She became cheerful, friendly, helpful, polite and very pleasant.

Her weight before the operation had been 4 st. 13 lb. It was up to 6 st. on her removal for convalescence. (She is 5 ft. 5½ in. in height.) She was eating extremely well. After three months of rehabilitation she was discharged home. Arrangements were made for her to return to her old employment, the firm being very willing to re-employ her. Ada started doing part-time, but is now working full-time. The employers, family and Ada herself are exceedingly contented with the 'cure' of her illness and her present state of health.

(d) Penelope, aged 63, was living in a small village where she worked as district nurse for twenty-seven years, before her retirement at the age of 60. She has her own home, is unmarried and is living on a pension. Her personality prior to her illness was reported to be very reserved, but she was able to make friends easily and enjoy company. She was predominantly a happy person and free from alternating moods, never really depressed, excessively conscientious and characteristically house-proud. Religion has played a large part in her life. She has taught at the Sunday school and is a staunch member of the church-going community.

The patient came from an affectionate, happy and healthy family. One great sorrow in her life had been the death of her brother when she was 27. She had been depressed and solitary as a result of this, but did not give up her work. Penelope worked for nineteen years as a domestic help before she could afford to train as a midwife.

The patient stated that she never had any sexual associations or interests. As she put it, 'my work satisfies me'. She never experienced any conscious regret regarding this, and has mixed equally well with men and women. Her life has, however, brought her into much more contact with women than with men.

About three years ago the symptoms started. These consisted of unpleasant ideas that kept coming into her mind. These ideas were entirely concerned with sex and swear-words, some of which Penelope did not realise she had ever heard. She became depressed and suicidal, complained of severe incapacitating headaches and felt that something had gone out of her life. She was constantly weeping and complaining, but managed to keep going and continued with her church work until she came into hospital. The prevailing expression of this small grey-haired woman was sad and worried.

Six months after her retirement—when her symptoms started—she had spent her day keeping the house clean, reading, seeing friends and knitting. As she felt bored she tried temporary work, doing her old job for one day a week and an occasional fortnight, and throughout the year was able to do this adequately.

At first she could get rid of her unpleasant thoughts when she concentrated on reading or writing. Gradually the thoughts intruded at all times, to the extent of making it difficult for her to carry on a conversation or listen to the wireless. This had become much worse during the last year and was now happening all the time. It prevented her from going to sleep at night, and occurred first thing in the morning; the content of these thoughts remained unchanged throughout. These visual imaginings and sexual words came into her mind in connection with innocent people and even children. She states, 'I can't say them; I have never said them; it's bad enough to have them inside me without saying them out loud.' Her depression increased, and she prayed to die, and felt that if she had not been a deeply religious person she would have made an end of it all. It seemed to her that if she had planned her life fully and if she had realised her need for constant activity her illness would never have happened.

Electric shock treatment was tried with no effect. As no other form of treatment was considered likely to help, it was then decided to carry out a leucotomy. After a unilateral right Rostral operation Penelope made a good recovery. In hospital she appeared less inhibited and in an elated mood. Improvement occurred gradually with regard to the obsessional thoughts. Five weeks after the operation she left hospital for a period of convalescence. On coming to out-patients after this, she was extremely happy with her condition, mentioning that everyone seemed kinder than before. She was brisk and bright, and remarked to the writer that the people she came into contact with appeared completely different since her operation. Penelope is now living with a sister in the West Country and it is reported that all continues well.

Note : The above case histories are based on the material in the medical folders. The writer's impressions have not been included except where explicitly stated. Examples of Barbara's and Simon's statements were presented in Appendix C.

APPENDIX E

A BRIEF REVIEW OF PREVIOUS
INVESTIGATIONS USING PSYCHOLOGICAL
TECHNIQUES

PSYCHOLOGICAL investigations into the effect of leucotomy are based on the psychiatric studies that preceded them. But as the special contribution of the work reported here is the objective measurement of personality changes following on the operation, no detailed review of psychiatric investigations will be attempted.

Comprehensive reviews and reports of psychiatric work have, however, been published by many writers, including the following: Freeman and Watts (1942) and Freeman (1950), Fleming (1944) and (1950), Walker (1944), Klebanoff (1945), Hebb (1945), Brody and Moore (1946), Rylander and Sjöqvist (1946), Garmany (1948), Henderson (1948), Ström-Olsen et al. (1943) and (1949), Stengel (1950), Greenblatt et al. (1950), Partridge (1950), Fernandes (1950) and Feiling (1951).

INTELLIGENCE AND INTELLECTUAL FUNCTIONING

In the study of the effect of leucotomy, considerably more reports of investigations using tests of intelligence than tests of temperament and character have been published, from which it is clear that certain aspects of intelligence are affected by the usual posterior operation of prefrontal leucotomy. The apparent absence of intellectual changes in some of these studies was due to the fact that a few of the investigators used psychotic subjects, whose pre-operative condition was so deteriorated in comparison with their normal intelligence level prior to their illnesses as to disguise the loss in intellectual aspects following on the operation, and not seldom to the fact that tests chosen measured those facets of intelligence which are unaffected by leucotomy. In some cases a more anterior incision was made, and this, as has been shown in Chapter IV, does not lead to a pronounced deficit in the intellectual aspects of personality. The pattern of change in intellectual function appeared to manifest itself best when a large battery of tests was used, such as in the Wechsler scale, and when the possibility existed of contrasting the behaviour on verbal and performance tests. Investigators using the Stanford Binet scale have shown a slight decrease in I.Q., which, however, has not reached the level of statistical significance (Ström-Olsen et al., 1943; Porteus and Kepner, 1944; Rylander, 1948; Yacorzynski et al., 1948).

Significant changes have been found in three investigations using the Wechsler scale (Koskoff et al., 1948; Malmo, 1948; Petrie, 1948c). These were carried out on seven, six and twenty patients respectively. The first group were cases of intractable pain and were retested three months after the operation. Losses tended to be greater on the verbal than on the performance scale in four investigations based on the scores of seven, twenty, two and one patients respectively (Koskoff et al., 1948; Petrie, 1948c; Yacorzynski et al., 1948; Jones, 1949).

Confirmation of a greater loss on verbal than on performance tests of intelligence comes from other sources than the Wechsler scale. Thus six cases were shown to lose on the Standard Binet vocabulary test, though not on other tests of intelligence (Malmo, 1948).

Performance Tests of Intelligence

It is of interest to report that in two investigations slight gains were found on performance tests (Koh's Blocks and Alexander's 'Pass Along' test), but they did not reach the level of significance (Hunt, 1942; Ström-Olsen et al., 1943). In an investigation of twenty-four chronic schizophrenics, a significant increase was, however, found on the Good-enough 'Draw a man' test (Jones, 1949).

There is also a report based on the performance of eleven chronic patients tested before and after the operation that a non-verbal perceptual test (Raven's Matrices) shows a slight but insignificant rise (Ström-Olsen et al., 1943).

Porteus Mazes

Those familiar with Porteus Maze tests will realise that an increase in impulsiveness, for example, will be likely to lower I.Q. scores. Because of these and various other differences which exist between the bulk of performance tests and that of Porteus, it is desirable to treat the maze results separately.

Porteus Mazes have been used by a number of workers and from the results there is evidence that this test is sensitive to changes following on leucotomy (Porteus and Kepner, 1944; Porteus and Peters, 1947; Petrie, 1948c; Porteus, 1950). Porteus points out that various investigations have shown that this maze test correlates more highly with some of the verbal tests of intelligence than with the performance tests. Unlike many of the performance tests, moreover, it is untimed and the quality of the manual performance does not gain marks in so far as the main I.Q. score is concerned. He also points out that the test appears to be a measure of personality as well as of intelligence and that it therefore is more sensitive to the type of change following on leucotomy than are many other tests.

There are two reports in the literature of investigations using Porteus Mazes which did not show a loss in I.Q. (Ström-Olsen *et al.*, 1943; Jones, 1949). These were carried out on eleven chronic patients and twenty-four schizophrenics respectively. In interpreting these results, however, it should be pointed out that Porteus has shown considerable practice effect in using these mazes on a control population, 21% improving on the second testing. This practice effect may be disguising some of the deficit in leucotomy patients.

The Work of Halstead

Halstead has suggested that there is a fundamental form of intelligence which is not measured by the standardised psychometric tests; he has called this 'Biological Intelligence'. He states that this consists of the four factors found in a factor analysis of intercorrelation between thirteen neuropsychological variables. The scores are those of fifty male patients who have had concussive types of head injury. He suggests that 'Biological Intelligence' is localised in the cortex (Halstead, 1947).

Some of the tests differentiate between lobectomy cases, where the whole of the frontal lobe has been removed, and other patients. His leucotomised patients, however, show no significant change on these tests after their operation. In spite of the absence of differences on these tests after leucotomy, Halstead thinks that 'Biological Intelligence' has its maximum representation in the frontal lobes, and suggests that it was already damaged in the patients who underwent leucotomy and therefore did not appear to be affected by the operation.

Two reviews of this work by Zangwill (1949) and Crown (1951) have suggested that these findings were not based on sufficient data and that the investigations so far have only shown that it is possible to differentiate, by a group of psychophysical and mental tests, between individuals who have no frontal lobes and those who have.

Investigations into Abstraction

Some work has been done which suggests that abstraction is affected by prefrontal leucotomy (Greenblatt et al., 1947; Yacorzynski et al., 1948; Malmo, 1948). Other workers suggest that there are no important changes on tests of abstract thinking (Kisker, 1944A; Jones, 1949).

Both the reported loss and absence of loss are, however, based on a wide variety of tests, some of which are purely of intelligence. Some tests do appear to involve the capacity to group to a criterion and these may be measures of the ability to abstract. Further research would be required to determine how consistently such results are found, and what interpretation should be ascribed to a loss on these tests.

REPORTS OF CHANGES IN TEMPERAMENT AND CHARACTER

Until recent years few investigations of changes in temperament and character as opposed to intelligence have been carried out on patients undergoing operations on the frontal lobes. This is surprising, as it was clear to the physicians that the changes following on prefrontal leucotomy were largely in the orectic sphere of personality.

There are a number of reports of studies dealing with the interpretation of Rorschach Ink Blots (Rapaport, 1946). Some slight quantitative changes have been demonstrated, but unfortunately there is little agreement between investigators as to what changes take place as a result of the operation (Kisker,

1944B; Jones, 1949). There is, however, in the work of Hunt (1942) some qualitative evidence of a decrease in neuroticism derived from the Rorschach tests.

An attempt was made to investigate the effect of leucotomy on the 'creative personality' (Hutton and Bassett, 1948). In this investigation the Rorschach records after the operation were compared with the records of other patients of similar diagnosis, social background and intelligence as the operated group. It was found that the operated group showed less originality and creative capacity according to the Rorschach records than the other patients. A multiple-choice Rorschach was also used on the same group. These results—combined with the clinical observation of lack of initiative, a tendency to live in the immediate present and to depend on the immediate environment for stimulation—also suggested to the authors that there might be a loss in creative activity after leucotomy.

The same conclusion is drawn from the patients' productions when they were asked to write a story introducing certain set sentences. The patients' stories, it is reported, tended to be brief and to report something read, heard or experienced. A small group also produced paintings after leucotomy and these were rated low for creative ability.

Some further investigations of this aspect have been carried out by Ashby and Bassett (1949) and a test of creative ability has been developed which requires the patient to add details to a painting. The performance of patients after the operation was compared with a group of psychotics and normal subjects. These results did not, however, provide evidence that creative ability is impaired by leucotomy.

An excellent review of psychometric studies of the effect of prefrontal leucotomy has been published by Crown (1951). He suggests that these findings on 'creative personality' are difficult to assess because patients were not examined before and after the operation, so that there is no evidence of a change in creative urge as a result of leucotomy.

A loss in the capacity for prolonged attention after leucotomy has been suggested as a result of another investigation (Robinson, 1946). This hypothesis was tested by 'deliberation' tests consisting of rhyme-making and simple mental arithmetic. These results, compared with that of a control group, suggested a definite intellectual deficit in the function which is called by this author 'prolonged attention'. A further investigation tended to confirm this hypothesis (Robinson *et al.*, 1949). In this study tests were used in which patients were required to disguise their handwriting and to write as slowly as possible. A test of speed of decision was also included. The author states that the common factor in these 'deliberation' tests is the capacity for prolonged attention and deliberativeness and that this is diminished after leucotomy. Crown (1951) states 'it is difficult to judge this experiment in isolation, as the significance of the results depends largely upon the results of research into a psychological nature of deliberativeness, if such a quality exists, and whether, if it exists, it can be validly measured by the test described.'

Another suggestion made by some workers (Babcock, 1947; Koskoff *et al.*, 1948) is that what they call 'basic efficiency' is affected by leucotomy. This conclusion is based on changes on tests of motor control, learning, perception and speed. These results were, however, based on six cases only.

By using the Bernreuter personality inventory on seven patients, a decrease in neuroticism was shown by Hunt (1942). In addition this inventory used on the same patients suggested a decrease in introversion.

In general it will be observed that most of the investigators had a very difficult task in attempting to detect personality changes following leucotomy, because the work had been carried out on groups of less than twenty individuals, and on deteriorated psychotics rather than neurotics who formed the great majority of the seventy patients discussed in the present work.

BIBLIOGRAPHY

ADRIAN, E. D. The aims of medicine. *Lancet,* **2**: 997, 1948.

ALCALDE, S. O. *Las Modernas Intervenciones Quirurgicas en Psiquiatra.* Madrid, 1947.

ANDERSON, A. L., and HANVIC, L. J. The psychometric localisation of brain lesions—the differential effect of frontal and parietal lesions. *J. Clin. Psychol.* **6**: 177, 1950.

ASHBY, W. R., and BASSETT, M. The effect of leucotomy on creative ability. *J. Ment. Sci.* **95**: 418, 1949.

BABCOCK, H. A case of anxiety neurosis before and after lobotomy. *J. Abnorm. (Soc.) Psychol.* **42**: 466, 1947.

BERLINER, F., MAYER-GROSS, W., BEVERIDGE, R. L., and MOORE, J. N. P. Prefrontal leucotomy. Report on 100 cases. *Lancet,* **2**: 325, 1945.

BOYD, D. A., and NIEL, W. Congenital universal indifference to pain. *Arch. Neurol. & Psychiat.* **61**: 402, 1949.

BRADY, M. Suggestibility and persistence in neurotics. *J. Ment. Sci.* **94**: 445, 1948.

BRAIN, W. R. The cerebral basis of consciousness. *Section of Neurol., Proc. R. Soc. Med.* **44**: 37, 1951.

BRICKNER, R. *The Intellectual Functions of the Frontal Lobes.* New York, The Macmillan Co., 1936.

BRODY, E., and MOORE, B. Prefrontal lobotomy; review of recent literature. *Conn. Med. J.* **10**: 409, 1946.

BRUNS, L. *Die Geschwülste des Nervensystems,* Berlin. 1897.

CAMERON, N. Reasoning regression and communication in schizophrenics. *Psychol. Monogr.* **50**: No. 1, 1938.

CATTELL, R. B. *A Guide to Mental Testing.* Univ. of London Press, 1936.

—— *Description and Measurement of Personality.* New York, Yonkers-on-Hudson, 1946A.

—— The riddle of perseveration: I, Disposition; II, Personality structure. *J. Personal.* **14**: 229, 1946B.

—— *Personality—a Systematic, Theoretical and Factual Study.* New York, McGraw-Hill Book Co., 1950.

——, and LUBORSKY, L. B. Personality factors in response to humour. *J. Abnorm. (Soc.) Psychol.* **42**: 402, 1947.

BIBLIOGRAPHY

CHAPMAN, W. P., ROSE, A. S., and SOLOMON, H. C. Measurements of heat stimulus producing motor withdrawal reaction in patients following frontal lobotomy. *Res. Nerv. Ment. Dis.* **27**: 754, 1948.

CLAUSEN, J., and KING, H. F. Determination of the pain thresholds of untrained subjects. *J. Psychol.* **30**: 299, 1950.

COHN, R. Electroencephalographic study of prefrontal lobotomy—a study of focal brain injury. *Arch. Neurol. & Psychiat.* **53**: 283, 1945.

CRITCHLEY, MACD. Speech iterations. *Post. Grad. Med. J.* **24**: 267, 1948.

—— Personal communication, 1950.

CROWN, S. Psychological changes following prefrontal leucotomy. *J. Ment. Sci.* **97**: 49, 1951.

CURETON, T. K., HUFFMAN, W. J., WELSER, L., KIREILIS, R. W., and LATHAM, D. E. Endurance of young men; analysis of endurance exercises and methods of evaluating motor fitness. *Monogr. Soc. Res. Child Develop.* **10**: No. 1, 284, 1945.

CURRAN, D., and GUTTMAN, E. *Psychological Medicine.* Edinburgh, E. & S. Livingstone, 1943.

DAX, E. C., and RADLEY SMITH, E. J. Early effects of prefrontal leucotomy on disturbed patients with mental illness of long duration. *J. Ment. Sci.* **89**: 182, 1943.

DERNER, G. F., ABORN, M., and CANTER, A. H. Reliability of the Wechsler-Bellevue sub-tests and scales. *J. Consult. Psychol.* **14**: 3, 1950.

EYSENCK, H. J. Types of personality; a factorial study of 700 neurotics. *J. Ment. Sci.* **90**: 851, 1944A.

—— States of high suggestibility and the neuroses. *Amer. J. Psychol.* **57**: 406, 1944B.

—— *Dimensions of Personality.* London, Kegan Paul, 1947.

—— Cyclothymia and schizothymia as a dimension of personality. *J. Personal.* **19**: 123, 1950.

——, and FURNEAUX, W. D. Primary and secondary suggestibility; an experimental and statistical study. *J. Exp. Psychol.* **35**: 485, 1945.

EYSENCK, M. D. Neurotic tendencies in epilepsy. *J. Neurol. Neurosurg. Psychiat.* **13**: 237, 1950.

FEILING, A. *Modern Trends in Neurology.* London, Butterworth & Co. Ltd., 1951.

FERNANDES, H. J. Anatamo-physiologie cérébrale et fonctions psychiques dans la leucotomie préfrontale. *Proc. Int. Cong. Psychiat.* **3**: Paris, 1950.

FLEMING, G. W. T. H. Prefrontal leucotomy. *J. Ment. Sci.* **90**: 486, 1944.
—— *Recent Progress in Psychiatry.* London, L. A. Churchill, 2nd edition, 1950.
FLUGEL, J. C. In discussion on leucotomy at Med. Sec. of Brit. Psychol. Soc., 1949.
FRANK, J. Clinical survey and results of 200 cases of prefrontal leucotomy. *J. Ment. Sci.* **92**: 497, 1946.
FRANKL, L., and MAYER-GROSS, W. Personality changes after prefrontal leucotomy. *Lancet,* **2**: 820, 1947.
FRANZ, S. I. On the functions of the cerebrum; the frontal lobes. *Arch. Psychol.* **1**: (No. 2), New York, Science Press. Quoted by King in Mettler, 1949.
FREEMAN, W. Psychosurgery. A. Neuropsychiatric aspects. *Progress Neurol. Psychiat.* **5**: 398, 1950.
——, and WATTS, J. W. *Psychosurgery: Intelligence, Emotion and Social Behaviour following Prefrontal Lobotomy for Mental Disorders.* London, Baillière, Tindall & Cox, 1942.
——, and —— Psychosurgery: an evaluation of 200 cases over seven years. *J. Ment. Sci.* **90**: 532, 1944.
——, and —— Schizophrenia in childhood; its modification by prefrontal lobotomy. *Dig. Neurol. Psychiat.* **15**: 202, 1947.
FREUDENBERG, R. K., GLEES, P., OBRADER, S., FOSS, B., and WILLIAMS, M. Experimental studies of frontal lobe functions in monkeys in relation to leucotomy. *J. Ment. Sci.* **96**: 143, 1950.
FRUCHTER, B. The nature of verbal fluency. *Educ. Psychol. Monogr.* **8**: 33, 1948.
GARMANY, G. Personality change and prognosis after leucotomy. *J. Ment. Sci.* **94**: 428, 1948.
GARRISON, M. Affectivity. In Mettler, F. A. *Selective Partial Ablation of the Frontal Cortex.* New York, Hoeber, Inc., 1949.
GIBBY, R. G. A preliminary survey of certain aspects of Form II of the Wechsler-Bellevue Scale compared to Form I. *J. Clin. Psychol.* **5**: 4, 1950.
GLEES, P., COLE, J., WHITTY, C. W. M., and CAIRNS, H. The effects of lesions in the cingular gyrus and adjacent areas in monkeys. *J. Neurol., Neurosurg. Psychiat.* **13**: 178, 1950.
GOLDSTEIN, K. The significance of the frontal lobes for mental performance. *J. Neurol. Psychopath.* **17**: 27, 1936.
GOLLA, F. R. Prefrontal leucotomy with reference to indications and results. *Proc. R. Soc. Med.* **29**: 443, 1946.
GORDON, R. A. An experiment correlating the nature of imagery with performance on a test of reversal of perspective. *Brit. J. Psychol.* **41**: 63, 1950.

BIBLIOGRAPHY

GREENBLATT, M., ARNOT, R. E., POPPEN, J. L. V., and CHAPMAN, W. P. Report on lobotomy studies at the Boston Psychopathic Hospital. *Amer. J. Psychiat.* **104**: 361, 1947.

———, ———, and SOLOMON, H. C. *Studies in Lobotomy*. New York, Grune & Stratton, Inc., 1950.

GUTTMAN, L. Rehabilitation after injuries to the spinal cord and cauda equina. *Brit. J. Phys. Med.* Vol. 19, **6**: 162, 1946.

HALSTEAD, W. C. *Brain and Intelligence*. University Chicago Press, 1947.

HAMISTER, R. C. Test and retest reliability of the Wechsler-Bellevue. *J. Consult. Psychol.* **13**: No. 1, 1949.

HARLOW, J. M. Passage of an iron rod through the head. *Boston M. & S. J.* **39**: 389, 1848.

HARROWER-ERIKSON, M. R. Personality changes accompanying cerebral lesions. I. Rorschach studies of patients with cerebral tumours. *Arch. Neurol. Psychiat.* **43**: 859, 1940.

HEBB, D. O. Man's Frontal Lobes: a critical review. *Arch. Neurol. Psychiat.* **54**: 10, 1945.

HENDERSON, D. Psychiatric hypothesis and practice. *J. Ment. Sci.* **94**: 394, 1948.

HIMMELWEIT, H. T. The intelligence vocabulary ratio as a measure of temperament. *J. Personal.* **14**: 93, 1945.

——— Speed of accuracy and work as related to temperament. *Brit. J. Psychol.* **36**: 132, 1946.

——— A comparative study of the level of aspiration of normal and neurotic persons. *Brit. J. Psychol.* **37**: 41, 1947.

———, DESAI, M., and PETRIE, A. An experimental investigation of neuroticism. *J. Personal.* **15**: 173, 1946.

———, and PETRIE, A. The measurement of personality in children; an experimental investigation of neuroticism. *Brit. J. Educ. Psychol.* **21**: Part 1, 9, 1951.

HULL, C. L. *Hypnosis and Suggestibility*. New York, Appleton Century. 1933.

HUNT, J. McV. *Personality and Behaviour Disorders*. New York, The Ronald Press Co., 1944.

HUNT, T. Intelligence and personality profile studies following pre-frontal lobotomy. In Freeman, W., and Watts, J. W., *Psychosurgery*. London, Baillière, Tindall & Cox, 1942.

HUTTON, E. L., and BASSETT, M. The effect of leucotomy on creative personality. *J. Ment. Sci.* **94**: 332, 1948.

ISRAELI, N. *Abnormal Personality and Time*. New York, Science Press Printing Co., 1936.

JACKSON, J. H. *Convulsive Seizures*. New York, 1890.

JACOBSEN, C. F. Studies of cerebral functions in primates. I. The function of the frontal association areas in monkeys. *Comp. Psychol. Monogr.* **13**: 1, 1936.

BIBLIOGRAPHY

JANET, P. *Les obsessions et la psychasthénie.* Paris, Alcan, 1903.

JONES, M. Responses to stress in neurotic patients. *J. Ment. Sci.* **94** : 392, 1948.

JONES, R. E. Personality changes in psychotics following prefrontal lobotomy. *J. Abnorm. (Soc.) Psychol.* **44**: 315, 1949.

JUNG, C. G. *Psychological Types.* London, Kegan Paul, 1923.

KISKER, G. W. Abstract and categorical behaviour following therapeutic brain surgery. *Psychosom. Med.* **6**: 146, 1944A.

—— The Rorschach analysis of psychotics subjected to neurosurgical interruption of the thalamo-cortical connections. *Psychiat. Quart.* **18**: 43, 1944B.

KLEBANOFF, S. G. General review and summary. Psychological changes in organic brain lesions and ablations. *Psychol. Bull.* **42**: 585, 1945.

KOSKOFF, Y. D., DENNIS, W., LAZOVIK, D., and WHEELER, E. T. The psychological effects of frontal lobotomy performed for the alleviation of pain. Section II. Changes in intellectual functions following frontal lobotomy. *Res. Publ. Ass. Nerv. Ment. Dis.* **27**: 741, 1948.

KRAYENBÜHL, H., and STOLL, W. Prefrontal leucotomy and topectomy for the relief of intractable pain. *Dig. Neurol. Psychiat.* **17**: 564, 1949.

LE BEAU, J. Localisation cérébrale de la conscience. *Revue Canadienne de Biologie,* **1**: No. 2, 134, 1942.

——, and PECKER, J. Études de certains formes d'agitation psychomatrice au cours de l'épilepsie et de l'arriération mentale, traitées par la topectomie péricalleuse antérieure bilatérale. *Estrait de La Semaine des Hôpitaux de Paris,* No. 33, 1950.

LURIA, A. R. *The Nature of Human Conflicts.* New York, Liveright, 1932.

McDOUGALL, W. *Outline of Abnormal Psychology.* London, Methuen & Co., 1926.

McKISSOCK, W. The technique of prefrontal leucotomy. *J. Ment. Sci.* **89**: 194, 1943.

—— Recent techniques in psychosurgery. Anglo-American Symposium, *Proc. R. Soc. Med.* Vol. 42, Supp., p. 13, 1949.

McLARDY, T., and MEYER, A. Anatomical correlates of improvement after leucotomy. *J. Ment. Sci.* **95**: 182, 1949.

MALMO, R. B. Psychological aspects of frontal gyrectomy and frontal lobotomy in mental patients. *Res. Publ. Ass. Nerv. Ment. Dis.* **27**: 537, 1948.

METTLER, F. A. (Ed.) *Selective Partial Ablation of the Frontal Cortex.* New York, Hoeber, Inc., 1949.

BIBLIOGRAPHY

MEYER, A. Anatomical lessons from prefrontal leucotomy. *Proc. Int. Cong. Psychiat.* **3**: 107, 1950.

——, and BECK, E. Neuropathological problems arising from prefrontal leucotomy. *J. Ment. Sci.* **91**: 411, 1945.

MONIZ, E. *Tentatives opératoires dans le traitement de certaines psychoses.* Paris, Masson & Cie, 1937.

MURRAY, H. A., *et al. Explorations in Personality.* New York, Oxford University Press, 1938.

NOBELE,——. *Annal. de méd. belge:* Férrier, Compte rendu, cited by H. Haeser, 1836. Fall einer bedeutenden Gehirnverletzung. *Schmidt's Jahrbücher,* **9**: 321, 1835.

ÖDEGÄRD, O. Report on 8th Congress of Scandinavian Psychiatrists in Copenhagen, Denmark, 1946. *Acta. Psychiat. Neurol.* **47**: 360, 1947.

OSMOND, H. An account of E.C.T. given to a patient with a tantalum plate in his skull. *J. Ment. Sci.* **97**: 381, 1951.

PARTRIDGE, M. A. *Prefrontal Leucotomy.* Oxford, Blackwell Scientific Publications, 1950.

PAVLOV, I. P. *Conditioned Reflexes and Psychiatry.* London, Lawrence & Wishart, 1941.

PENFIELD, W., and RASMUSSEN, T. *The Cerebral Cortex of Man. A Clinical Study of Localisation of Function.* New York, The Macmillan Co., 1950.

PETRIE, A. Repression and suggestibility as related to temperament. *J. Personal.* **16**: 445, 1948A.

—— The selection of medical students. *Lancet,* **2**: 325, 1948B.

—— Personality changes after prefrontal leucotomy. *Proc. 12th Int. Cong. Psychol.* Edinburgh, 1948C.

—— Preliminary report of changes after prefrontal leucotomy. *J. Ment. Sci.* **95**: 449, 1949A.

—— Personality changes after prefrontal leucotomy. Report II. *Brit. J. Med. Psychol.* **22**: 200, 1949B.

—— Anglo-American Symposium. *Proc. R. Soc. Med.* Vol. 42, Supp., p. 39, 1949C.

—— The application of mental tests to clinical psychiatry. *Int. Cong. Psychiat.* Paris, 1950A.

—— Psychological investigations and cerebral anatomy. *Int. Cong. Psychiat.* Paris, 1950B.

—— Preliminary report of changes after prefrontal leucotomy. Personality changes after prefrontal leucotomy. *Dig. Neurol. Psychiat.* **18**: 474, 1950C.

—— A comparison of the psychological effects of two different types of incision on the frontal lobes. *Proc. 13th Int. Cong. Psychol.,* Stockholm, 1951.

PETRIE, A. and POWELL, M. B. Personality and nursing—an investigation into selection tests for nurses. *Lancet*, **1**: 363, 1950.

——, and —— Selection of nurses in England. *J. Appl. Psychol.* **35**: No. 1, 1951.

PICHOT, P. *Les Testes Mentaux à Psychiatrie.* (1) *Instruments et Méthodes.* Paris, Press Université de France, 1949.

PORTEUS, S. D. *The Maze Test and Mental Differences.* Vincland, N. J., Smith, 1933.

—— Medical applications of the Maze Test. *Med. J. Aust.* **1**: 550, 1944.

—— Thirty-five years' experience with the Porteus Maze. *J. Abnorm. (Soc.) Psychol.* **45**: No. 2, 396, 1950.

——, and KEPNER, R. D. Mental changes after bilateral prefrontal lobotomy. *Genet. Psychol. Monogr.* **29**: 3, 1944.

——, and PETERS, H. N. Psychosurgery and test validity. *J. Abnorm. (Soc.) Psychol.* **42**: 473, 1947.

RAPAPORT, D. *Diagnostic Psychological Testing.* Chicago, The Year Book Publishers, 1946.

REES, W. L. L. Body build, personality and neurosis in women. *J. Ment. Sci.* **96**: 426, 1950.

——, and EYSENCK, H. J. A factorial study of some morphological and psychological aspects of human constitution. *J. Ment. Sci.* **91**: 8, 1945.

RESEARCH ASSOCIATION IN NERVOUS AND MENTAL DISEASE. The Frontal Lobes. Vol. 27. Baltimore, Williams & Wilkins, 1948.

RITCHIE RUSSELL, W. Functions of the frontal lobes. *Lancet*, **1**: 356, 1948.

ROBINSON, M. F. What price lobotomy? *J. Abnorm. (Soc.) Psychol.* **41**: 421, 1946.

——, FREEMAN, W., and WATTS, J. W. Personality changes after psychosurgery. *Dig. Neurol. Psychiat.* **17**: 558, 1949.

ROSENZWEIG, S. The experimental measurement of types of reaction to frustration. In Murray, H. A., *et al.*, *Explorations in Personality.* New York, Oxford University Press, 1938.

——An outline of frustration theory. In J. McV. Hunt, *Personality and the Behaviour Disorders.* New York, The Ronald Press Co., 1944.

——, and SARASON, S. An experimental study of the triadic hypothesis. *Charact. & Pers.* **11**: 1, 1942.

RYANS, D. G. The measurement of persistence. *Psychol. Bull.* **36**: 715, 1939.

RYLANDER, G. *Personality Changes after Operations on the Frontal Lobes: A Clinical Study of 32 Cases.* London, Oxford University Press, 1939.

BIBLIOGRAPHY

RYLANDER, G. Mental changes after excision of cerebral tissue. *Acta. Psychiat. et Neurol.* **25**: 5, 1943.

—— Personality analysis before and after frontal lobotomy. *Res. Publ. Ass. Nerv. Ment. Dis.* **27**: 691, 1948.

——, and SJÖQVIST, O. Prefrontal lobotomy in mental diseases. *Nord. Med.* **29**: 557, 1946.

SIMPSON, R. C., and BARNES, H. The incidence of obsessional traits occurring in 100 consecutive admissions to Broadmoor, with a control series of 100 consecutive admissions to a Neurosis Centre. Personal communication, 1951.

SLORACH, J. Bullet wound through both frontal lobes with recovery. *Lancet*, **1**: 1331, 1951.

STENGEL, E. Studien über die Bezeihung zwichen Geistesstörung und Sprächstörung. *Monatschr. Psychiat. Neurol.* **95**: 129, 1937.

—— On learning a new language. *Int. J. Psycho-Anal.* **20**: 471, 1939.

—— A follow-up investigation of 330 cases treated by prefrontal leucotomy. *Dig. Neurol. Psychiat.* **18**: 623, 1950.

STRÖM-OLSEN, R., LAST, S. L., and BRODY, M. B. Results of prefrontal leucotomy in 30 cases of mental disorder. *J. Ment. Sci.* **89**: 165, 1943.

——, and TOW, P. MacD. Late social results of prefrontal leucotomy. *Lancet*, **1**: 87, 1949.

TERMAN, L. M., and MERRILL, M. A. *Measuring Intelligence.* London, Harrap, 1937.

TIFFIN, J. *Industrial Psychology.* New York, Prentice Hall, Incorp., 1946.

TOW, P. MacD. *Psychological Changes after Isolation of the Prefrontal Area.* Ph.D. Thesis, London University, 1951.

TURNER, O. A. Growth and development of the cerebral cortical pattern in man. *Arch. Neurol. Psychiat.* **59**: 1, 1948.

—— Some data concerning the growth and development of the cerebral cortex in man. II. Post-natal growth changes in the cortical surface area. *Arch. Neurol. Psychiat.* **64**: 378, 1950.

WALKER, A. E. Psychosurgery; collective review. *Int. Abstr. Surg.* **78**: 1, 1944.

WECHSLER, D. *Measurement of Adult Intelligence.* Baltimore, Williams & Wilkins, 1944.

—— *The Wechsler-Bellevue Intelligence Scale Form II.* Manual for administering and scoring the test. New York, The Psychological Corporation, 1946.

WELT, L. Über Charakterveränderungen des Menschen infolge von Läsionen des Stirnhirns. *Deutsches Arch. f. klin. Med. von Ziemssen.* **42**: 339, 1888.

BIBLIOGRAPHY

WOLFF, H. G., and GOODELL, H. The relation of attitude and suggestion to the perception and reaction to pain. *Res. Publ. Ass. Nerv. Ment. Dis.* **23**: 434, 1943.

YACORZYNSKI, G. K., BOSHES, B., and DAVIS, L. Psychological changes produced by frontal lobotomy. *Res. Publ. Ass. Nerv. Ment. Dis.* **27**: 642, 1948.

YAHN, M. Mattos Pimenta & Afonso Sette Junior, *Psychosurgery.* Lisbon, 1949.

ZANGWILL, O. L. Review: Brain and intelligence: a quantitative study of the frontal lobes. By W. C. Halstead in *Quart. J. Exp. Psychol.* **1**: 147, 1949.

INDEX OF NAMES

SUBJECT INDEX

SUBJECT INDEX

SUBJECT INDEX

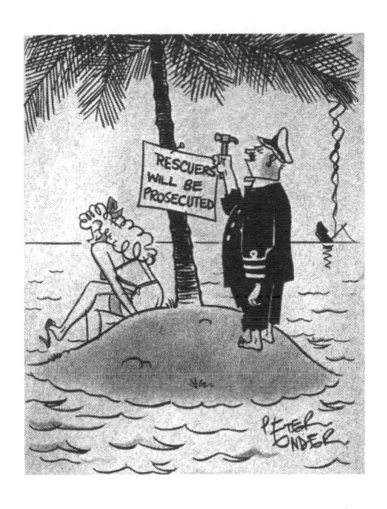

TYPE OF JOKE FOUND MORE AMUSING

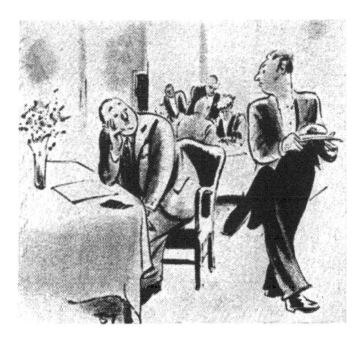

'You might tell them in the cloakroom to put moth balls in my things.'

TYPE OF JOKE FOUND LESS AMUSING

[*face page* 30